The
Models'
Way to Beauty,
Slenderness,
and
Glowing
Health

by
Oleda Baker
with
Bill Gale

Special Photographs by
Richard Hochman

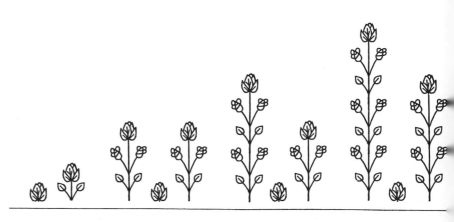

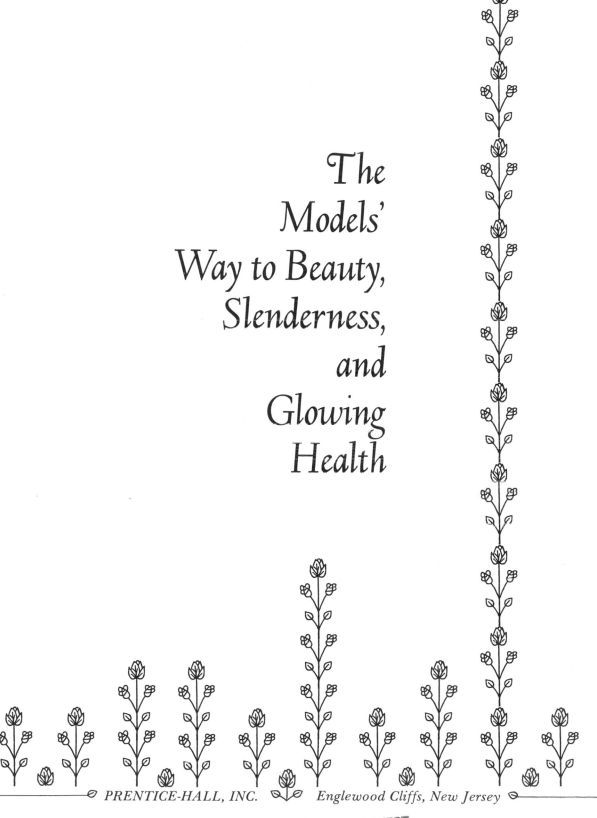

The
Models'
Way to Beauty,
Slenderness,
and
Glowing
Health

PRENTICE-HALL, INC. Englewood Cliffs, New Jersey

The Models' Way to Beauty, Slenderness, and Glowing Health
by Oleda Baker with Bill Gale
Copyright © 1973 by Oleda Baker
Special Photographs by Richard Hochman

Printed in the United States of America

Prentice-Hall International, Inc., London
Prentice-Hall of Australia, Pty. Ltd., North Sydney
Prentice-Hall of Canada, Ltd., Toronto
Prentice-Hall of India Private Ltd., New Delhi
Prentice-Hall of Japan, Inc., Tokyo

Library of Congress Cataloging in Publication Data

Baker, Oleda
    The models' way to beauty, slenderness, and glowing
health.

    1. Beauty, Personal. 2. Hygiene. 3. Models,
Fashion. I. Title.
RA778.B214   646.7   72-7214
ISBN 0-13-586073-3

To my husband,

who encouraged me to write this book . . .

Drawings by Onalee Fox.

Acknowledgments:

The author gratefully acknowledges permission to use recipes provided by Knox Gelatine, Inc., and Kretschmer Wheat Germ Products.

Introduction

Scene: A penthouse on Manhattan's East Side. A river view, with wall-to-wall carpeting and a crush of wall-to-wall people. The so-called Beautiful People.

Time: The mid-sixties.

Mood: Gay. And why not? There were scads of interesting men, berry-colored from weekends of golf, swimming, and sailing in the sun . . . and as the hostess, I had seen to it that they outnumbered the girls by a ratio of perhaps two to one. I was contentedly sipping a glass of white wine, and snubbing the delicious hors d'oeuvres in favor of the delicious conversation that Ping-Ponged around the room. Suddenly, as often happens at big parties, I found myself in conversation with one man . . . .

" . . . And you would be our Food, Fashion, and Beauty Editor," he was saying, assuming that I had heard what preceded this. I hadn't. So he repeated it. In capsule, this was the story: New York was then in the throes of a citywide newspaper strike and the unions had agreed that his East Side weekly could become a daily for the duration of the strike. Ergo: an immediate need for someone capable of putting out a two-page spread, five days a week, on food, fashion, and beauty. Would I be that someone?

"But why *me*?" I asked, scanning the room full of beautiful girls.

"Because I understand you have a five-year-old son and you look nineteen. You must know something a lot of other women don't."

Naturally I said I would do it. (How could I refuse after that?) And so for the next three months I worked perhaps harder than I ever have in my life. But I relished the challenge. And somehow I did manage to fill those two pages five days a week thanks to the generosity of my friends—other models—who clued me in to their beauty and diet secrets and their fashion know-how. It was during those hectic weeks that I *really* came to appreciate what a vast treasure of fascinating information we models accumulate as part of our profession.

Well, I was recently reminiscing with my husband about my "crash" career as a newspaper editor when he said, "You know, you should write a book." And since he's authored some eight books himself, I thought about it seriously . . . slept on the idea . . . and next morning, before breakfast, slipped downstairs, rolled a sheet of paper into our His 'n Her portable, and began this book.

I think you'll benefit from it and enjoy it. For once again I've enlisted the aid of my model friends whose glamorous faces and sleek, flat-tummied figures help sell everything from hair sprays and sable coats, to low-calorie salad dressings and high-priced sports cars.

So come with me behind the scenes, and let me show you what New York models do to get and keep our in-demand faces and figures.

Turn this page and step into our world—and by the time you turn the last page, I guarantee you'll look and feel like a *new* woman!

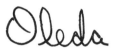

Contents

The
Models'
Way to Beauty,
Slenderness,
and
Glowing
Health

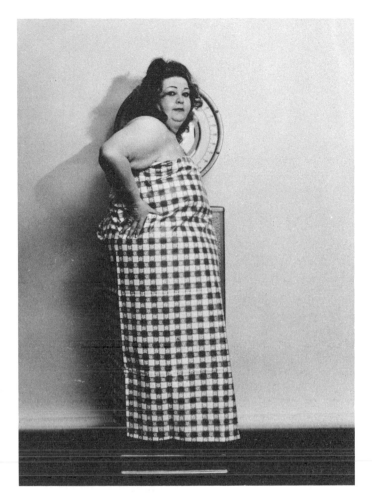
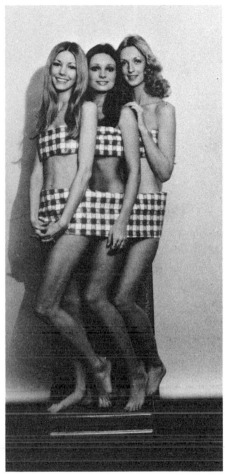

Wrapped in a tablecloth (with not an inch to spare), Pearl Yampolsky weighs in at 380 pounds. Wrapped (just barely) in snips of the same tablecloth, models Jo Anna McCarthy, Wendy August, and Kathy Jackson weigh in together at a grand total of 340 pounds. Now honestly, which size do you prefer?

CHAPTER · 1

"I Can't Lose
Weight Because..."

... Obesity runs in my family

Well, no better time than *now* to make it stop! Granted, obesity does run in some families, but that doesn't mean you have to sit back and accept your overweight as a kind of family curse. More than likely it's simply the result of careless or naïve eating habits and far too little physical activity—lazy habits passed on from generation to generation. Isn't it about time you refused to accept your legacy?

... I love food too much to starve myself

Do you think that makes you unique? I positively adore food! And I never, but never, starve myself. Yet I weigh the same today as I did when I started modeling more than ten years ago. Marlene Dietrich loves food, too, and I understand she's a fabulous cook as well. So I'm afraid you'll have to find another excuse to hide behind—this one's far too feeble.

... Dieting would make me nervous, irritable

Sheer nonsense! It's just the other way around. Diet properly and you'll not only look better, but you'll eat better than you probably have in years. And as those pounds melt away, you'll positively bubble with happiness!

... Dieting would make me look haggard

There is scarcely a New York model who didn't have to shed at least five to ten pounds (sometimes a lot more) before a model agency offered her a contract. And you can be sure the purpose was to make her look so divine she might one day become a *super* model

16

earning an annual six-figure income. Hags don't qualify, but fine-boned girls with smooth skin and flat tummies do—especially if they also have the energy of a topflight athlete.

. . . I'm too old to start dieting

Really? My mother, past sixty, recently dieted away fourteen pounds. Slim and vivacious, she looks sensational! And what does "too old" mean today, anyway? Actress Merle Oberon recently said: "Today we see the results of good diet, exercise, etc., in people who ten years ago would have been considered on the shelf. 'Middle age' is moving up to sixty!" And yes, I think of Lady Mendl, about whom I used to read when I was a schoolgirl in Florida. A famous international hostess and bright personality, she was still doing headstands each morning when she was in her eighties. Cecil Beaton called her "a factory of chic," and nutritionist Gaylord Hauser attributed her perfect figure to her habit of *under*eating always. This fascinating woman who lived a full, exciting life until her death at the age of ninety-plus said of herself, "The longer I live, the more I realize that it is never too late to learn." So toss away your inhibitions and start learning how to diet. It's never too late!

. . . My husband likes me this way

He does? In that case, he's either being overly kind (solicitous might be another way of putting it), or he's overweight himself, or he's simply telling a big fat lie! Look at your wedding picture, and then look into a full-length mirror. Be honest. Do *you* really prefer you overweight? Of course you don't! (And neither does he.) So let's bring back the girl he married.

Now, if overweight isn't your problem, then use this book to learn how to maintain your ideal weight. Let it show you how to add not so much as a single pound though you add five, ten, twenty, even thirty candles to your birthday cake. The fatalistic (lazy) attitude that middle-aged spread is an inevitable companion to middle age was long ago disproved by some of the world's most famous women who have absolutely refused to surrender their slim figures and youthful vitality.

17

Back in the thirties, for instance, when her husband was our Ambassador to the Court of St. James, raven-haired Rose Kennedy, then the mother of nine, was so strikingly slender and lovely that one evening as she entered a crowded ballroom, a well-known British diplomat was heard to remark, "Looking at her restores my faith in the stork." Almost thirty years later, on the occasion of John Fitzgerald Kennedy's Inaugural Ball, Rose Kennedy wore one of the classically beautiful evening gowns made for her during that period in England—her physical measurements not having changed one whit in the intervening years!

Glamorous Gloria Swanson at seventy-plus still looks pencil-slim and dainty in a pair of tailored pants—a feat some women half her age can't manage.

Joan Crawford, now in her sixties, weighs the same as she did forty years ago. "I'm a scale-watcher," she says, confiding that she weighs in every morning—making it as much a morning ritual as brushing her teeth.

And I don't know who was responsible for the moss-covered cliché that Latin women bloom early and fade early, but whoever that misguided creature was, I only wish he could have been with me the day I spied the fabulous Dolores Del Rio shopping in Saks Fifth Avenue. Past sixty, this exquisitely boned beauty in a face revealing turban and dramatic cape looked positively breathtaking!

So if you're past forty and slim, rejoice in the fact that you can remain slim and exciting for a lifetime. If you're overweight—no matter what your age—decide right now that you'll no longer tolerate so much as an extra pound to come between you and perfection. For it's never too late to learn to diet—and never too early to start.

This book is dedicated to the woman who would like to experience every woman's favorite fantasies:

> . . . To go to her high-school reunion and have every
> woman there look at her with envy.
> . . . To have her man scan a roomful of attractive women
> and then bring his eyes back to her—proud and loving.
> . . . To have her thirteen-year-old daughter come to her
> for beauty advice.
> . . . To be over forty and have a salesclerk offhandedly
> call her "Miss."

. . . To see a figure-revealing swimsuit and buy it—confident that she'll do it justice and vice versa.

In other words, unless I've misjudged you (and the fact that you've picked up this book and are reading it proves I haven't), this book is dedicated to a woman very much like YOU!

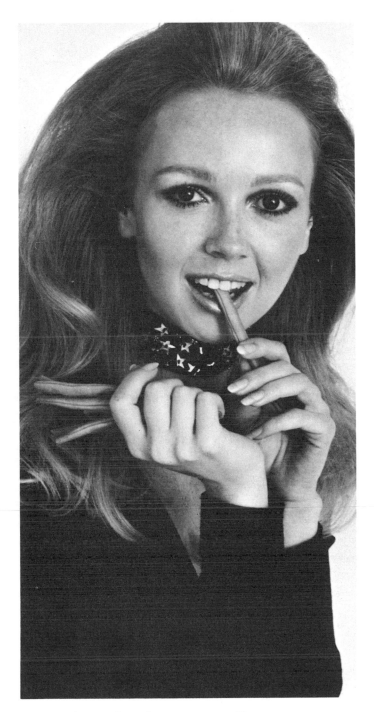

Penny James loves to munch on raw string beans. Once you've worked up your enthusiasm for dieting, you'll find there's something about a crunchy bean—and all the jaw action that goes into eating it—that tames a sudden urge to eat.

CHAPTER · 2

Enthusiasm—
Getting It and
Holding On to It

The inimitable Elizabeth Arden had a motto: ENTHUSIASM CAN CONQUER THE WORLD! Now, you might think that's a bit much, but enthusiasm is charmingly contagious, *and* absolutely essential to the launching of any worthwhile project—in this case, the new YOU! So it's important that you initiate your diet with positively bubbling enthusiasm. And why shouldn't you feel that way? You're about to start on what is going to prove to be one of the most gratifying experiences any woman can have.

Dr. Theodore Isaac Rubin, a psychiatrist and writer with a unique approach to what he calls "girth" control, stresses how necessary it is for the dieter to maintain an optimistic attitude. Dr. Rubin is convinced that *hopelessness* is the second biggest enemy of the dieter. The first? Dr. Rubin calls it *self-hate.* Together he sees them as traps used to maintain the *status quo*: FAT.

It would be childish, of course, to expect results overnight, but *do* expect results. Plan for the great day when you're going to be the perfect YOU. Meantime, however, live in the present. After all, anyone who has a sticky habit must learn to *un*learn it day by day. Your habit is overeating. So enjoy your new diet, understand what it is doing for you, and be true to it every day. But, keep the corners of your eyes trained on tomorrow and the day after tomorrow and the day after that, when you're going to look and feel slimmer, younger, and infinitely more attractive.

There are literally scads of ways to set yourself up so that you get the maximum out of your dieting adventure. Perhaps we models are experts in this area. Wander into Wilhelmina's Madison Avenue office almost any day, and you'll find a knot of girls with their heads together, deep in conversation. Discussing what? Men? Clothes? A creamy new mascara? A sensational new moisturizer that's light as a soufflé? Rarely. More often than not they're discussing their diets.

Not diets to lose weight (they've already done that), but the vim 'n vigor type diets they're following to maintain their ideal weight and overall good looks. For once you've dieted successfully you'll never want to stop. You'll have learned so much about nutrition, and developed such a healthy respect for your body, that you'll find it exciting to sample new dishes and improvise new menus—while maintaining your ideal weight. Suddenly your taste buds are "educated," and almost intuitively you find yourself able to eat what you want when you want, without gaining so much as an ounce. *You* are in control of your body, and food is now an ally rather than an enemy. It fills you up, but never out. Your tummy is flat, your hips are slim, you exude self-confidence and have energy to spare. You appear to breeze through the day, *every* day.

Sounds almost too good to be true? You'll discover it's true, every lovely bit of it. In fact, I envy you that day in your diet (and it will come before you're even halfway to your goal) when you feel different. Lighter. Freer. Your clothes are suddenly a little loose around the waist. You reach for something and your hand is there— almost before you realize it. Practically everything you do seems easier, more natural. You can't resist stealing a glance at yourself every time you pass a mirror. You can't help but smile at your own reflection. You and that woman in the mirror share a delicious secret that soon everyone will know. But for now it's all yours, and it's *delightful!*

In short, dieting can be fun. You can make it one of the happiest of adventures. And here are just a few of the ways models I know have kept it that way from optimistic start to glorious finish:

Be a Flamboyant Calorie Counter

If you and your doctor have decided to put you on a diet that calls for counting calories, become the most efficient, most turned-on calorie counter of all time! Start out by investing in a collection of calorie charts. They're almost always palm size and inexpensive enough so that you can afford a collection without feeling extravagant. The best of them not only list foods and their caloric content, but give you scratch paper so you can tally up a meal before you even pick up your fork. All in all, there's something reassuring about

23

a calorie chart, and I suggest you position yours strategically here, there, and everywhere. These cheery little diet helpers work like friendly porpoises, nudging you out of the dangerous waters which, in the diet season, are wherever temptation lies waiting in the form of a gooey dessert or rich sauce.

> . . . Tuck one into the frame of the mirror around your medicine chest, where it will greet you each morning as you reach for the toothpaste.
> . . . Play it cool and tape one inside the door of your refrigerator.
> . . . Tape another one inside the door of your clothes closet where all those soon-to-be-altered fashions are hanging.
> . . . Tape still another one on the wall just above your shower. And stare up at it and SMILE—as you suds a figure that's growing slimmer every day.
> . . . Slip one into your pocketbook, and make absolutely certain you're never without it when dining out.

Decorate Your Pantry

Divide its contents into two camps: the low-calorie foods and the high-calorie foods. Once that's done, start decorating. Perhaps a go-ahead green for the low-calorie shelf and a STOP, proceed-with-caution red for the high-calorie shelf.

And for good measure, you might consider decorating the interior of the pantry doors with clippings snipped from magazines and newspapers. "Stylish stouts" on one side, sleek models on the other. I know one model who had Maria Callas working for her in the kitchen via two magazine photos pasted on the inside of the refrigerator door. One showed La Callas rehearsing in Milan some twenty years ago—a 200-pound girl straining the boundaries of a long-sleeved sweater and rumpled-looking skirt. The other photo was the Maria Callas of the 1960s—looking svelte and cool in a skinny linen sheath aboard the Onassis yacht, with the skipper himself pouring her a glass of champagne.

Tricia Kinney, a pert young model, decorates the inside cover of

24

her portfolio with a full-color cartoon of Porky Pig—a whimsical reminder to bypass the malted milk bar on her way home.

Have a Weigh-In

You've heard of a Love-In. A Sit-In. Why not inaugurate a Weigh-In? Schedule it for the same day, some hour, every week. (Be sure it's the *same hour,* for weight does fluctuate during the course of the day. The ideal time for me, I've found, is as soon as I rise in the morning.) Of course, this doesn't mean you don't step on your scale every day, rain or shine. It's just that your Weigh-In Day is a *special* occasion—the day you toast your progress with a frosty glass of skim milk and dutifully note your poundage on the graph taped to the wall just above the scale. That graph of yours will prove a fantastic morale builder! The more you lose, the sharper its line will dip and the higher your spirits will soar. An upside-down graph like that would drive a businessman mad, but you'll adore being in the red!

If you have a friend who's also dieting, why not make it a duet on Weigh-In Day? Better yet, make it a friendly competition. At so much per pound.

Keep a Photo Album of Your Progress

Have your co-conspirator snap a picture of you at each weigh-in. Put each one in an album with the date clearly marked below—with, of course, your poundage. After a few weeks you'll see for yourself the change that's gradually taking place in you. By the time the last photo's been pasted in the album, what a merry cavalcade of before-and-after shots you'll have!

Think About Food

Tanya Leveau, an exotic beauty, did just that and it revolutionized her eating habits.

When Hong Kong-born Tanya married her handsome husband, Dominique, she weighed 115 pounds. Too much poundage, she decided, for her tiny frame, especially when matched to a whippet-slim Frenchman with, as she puts it, "not one fat molecule in his body."

So Tanya proceeded to convince herself that she didn't want any food that "would make me ugly." "I thought about what I was eating when I was eating it. I thought about mashed potatoes, for instance. I ate slowly and concentrated, and in my mind's eye they became like a solid weight. How *pulpy!* I lost my appetite for mashed potatoes and sold myself instead on leafy green vegetables. And so it went like that until I no longer had any desire for fattening foods." In her own words, she became a sensible, moderate eater.

In exactly five months' time Tanya slipped from 115 to 100 pounds, which is absolute perfection for her. Small-boned, slender yet daintily rounded, Tanya has one of the most beautiful, most graceful figures imaginable.

You might apply this same psychology—in reverse—to the foods you eat while dieting. Eat slowly, really *taste* those healthy, low-calorie foods. Feel their light texture. Where possible, let the food melt on your tongue. *Weightless.* Appreciate how this delicious food is nourishing you while helping you become slim. Be content in the knowledge that at last you're eating sensibly, healthfully, and toward a most worthwhile goal—a slimmer, healthier, happier you.

Make Mealtime a Happy Time

A serene, relaxed atmosphere at mealtime is always important, but never more so than when you're dieting. You simply must never feel that you're denying yourself. Therefore, make every effort to make mealtime a gracious occasion—even when you're all by yourself. *Never,* for example, allow a grocery jar or container on your table. You are your own guest and should be served properly.

Though I may lunch alone, I always set the table properly—the napkin in place, a bowl of fruit or flowers cheering up the center of the table. And I eat slowly—as you must. Never permit any meal to be rushed. For the more slowly you eat, the more you chew—and the less food you seem to need.

It's also important psychologically to fill the table. I find there's something quite depressing about a dining table with only one or two dishes on it. It's much too Spartan-looking. So even when I'm alone

26

and having a light luncheon that's really nothing more than what I call a "big nibble," I see to it that the table looks full: a big bowl of fresh fruit; a dish of chilled celery sticks; another dish of carrot sticks, and on and on. Colorful things to look at. Nice things to nibble on. When I'm simply having a sandwich, I put each of the ingredients on a separate dish and add a tray of radishes and condiments.

Determine now to make each meal a happy, gracious occasion, and I promise you that you'll never feel deprived at any time during your diet.

Buy a Bikini

Tuck it away in a drawer. Buy a glamorous dress in the size you want to be and hang it in your closet. Mark both "NOT TO BE OPENED UNTIL I WEIGH_____POUNDS." Talk about incentive! You've made a statement, you see. You've actually invested in your future, your *immediate* future. What more positive way to show your optimism!

Judy Brown, a 5'7" green-eyed beauty with mahogany-colored hair, decided she wanted a more sophisticated look. She felt the time had come for her to graduate from a teen magazine cover girl to more the *Cosmopolitan* type. After a visit to her doctor, Judy began a high-protein diet and in one season slipped from 125 to 105 pounds or, in model terminology, from the Junior to Junior Miss category. Midway in her diet—at the 113-pound mark—Judy splurged on a fabulous chiffon frock from famous designer Sarmi. It was the most expensive gown she'd ever bought. Not in the size she was, of course, but the size she was planning to be—a slip of a girl with a *22-inch waist!* Came spring and she wore her Sarmi chiffon for the first time, and Judy still recalls that evening as one of the most glamorous of her life.

Perhaps now you understand better what I mean when I say I *envy* you the experience you're about to have.

Your diet should be fitted to your way of life. If you like to snack, take a tip from Ingrid Drechsler, who prefers celery at snack time, consuming a mere 6 calories per stalk.

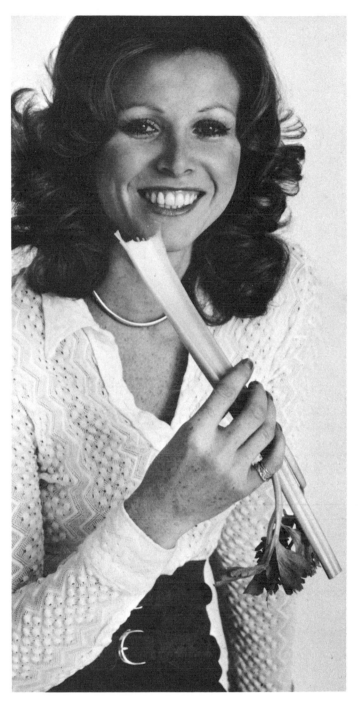

CHAPTER · 3

Choosing the
Diet Tailor-Made
for You

No two women—not even identical twins—are exactly alike. So the diet that's ideal for one may not be effective for the other. And with literally dozens of diets to choose from, why take potluck? Make absolutely certain that you select the diet that is ideally suited to your temperament, your metabolism, and your personal life-style.

The very first thing you do, of course, is to consult your physician. But I suggest you do your homework *before* you enter his inner sanctum. Play the comparison shopper. Bone up on some of the classic diets you have the pleasure of choosing from.

Here are just a few—enough, however, to prove beyond any doubt that dieting today can be an adventure in eating!

THE LOW-CARBOHYDRATE DIET: One of its most attractive rules is that you MUST eat *six times a day*. So much, then, for the old wives' tale that dieting spells deprivation.

But let's start at the very beginning. What are carbohydrates?

Carbohydrates are sugars and starches that supply your body with energy. They are measured by the gram. And the secret of a low-carbohydrate diet is that you limit yourself to a daily intake of no more than 60 grams, the rationale being that your body will then call upon its own fat—stored-up carbohydrates—for energy. Result: you lose weight, often at the sensible, eye-pleasing rate of three pounds a week! This diet, by the way, has earned the plaudits of many doctors who cast carbohydrates in the role of villain in the matter of heart and circulatory diseases.

Another perfectly delicious thing about this diet is that some of the most mouth-watering foods contain *no grams at all.* Roasted chicken, for example. A minute steak, fried or broiled. Roast loin of pork. Porterhouse steak. Roast leg of lamb. A martini cocktail adds up to a mere 0.3 grams—hardly worth mentioning. So you see, you certainly don't suffer on a low-carbohydrate diet.

30

Heather Hazell, one of our glamorous models shed ten pounds this way. "I weighed 130 in 1968 and my clients screamed all over the place!" recalls Heather, a topflight fashion show model whose clients include Givenchy, Elizabeth Arden, Christian Dior, and Maximilian, the posh furrier who whips up sumptuously furry creations like Russian broadtail suits and mink ski parkas. Now, a suddenly overweight model *might* pass muster in a photographer's studio posing for head shots, but she simply wouldn't be permitted to put one Gucci pump out on a fashion runway, where one pound is tragic—but TEN pounds are catastrophic, what with the aristocracy of the fashion press gaping up at you, often close enough to reach out and touch you. There's positively no escape. No flattering camera angles. No trick lighting. *Nothing.* You're slim, or else.

Here's a one-day menu from a low-carbohydrate diet, and I all but lick my lips as I type it:

BREAKFAST   *Grams*

½ cup puffed wheat (unsweetened) 4.8

   with 4 tablespoons light cream 2.4

   and 1 teaspoon confectioner's sugar 2.7

2-egg cheese omelette 9

   cooked in 2 tablespoons butter 2

3 slices of bacon, fried or broiled 3

                                          total   11.3

MID-MORNING

¾ cup bouillon, on the rocks 0

Sardines, canned in oil 0

4 tablespoons chived cottage cheese 1.6

   sprinkled with 4 pecans, chopped 9

                                          total   2.5

(It's already noon, and you've only consumed 13.8 grams!)

LUNCHEON

1 spritzer (3½ ounces dry white wine and club soda) 5

1 can tuna 0

   mixed with 2 tablespoons mayonnaise 1

   and ½ stalk celery, diced 1.0

½ medium tomato, sliced 3.5

2 saltines 5.8

   topped with 1 ounce bleu cheese spread 1.9

31

LUNCHEON (cont'd.)   *Grams*

2 chocolate wafer cookies	5.2
1 cup plain tea	.4
with ½ teaspoon lemon juice added	.2
total	18.6

MIDDAY

¾ cup jellied consomme	.0
topped with 2 tablespoons sour cream	1.0
and onion salt	.0
total	1.0

DINNER

1 spritzer	.5
Minute steak, sautéed	.0
in 2 tablespoons butter	.2
topped with pan juice	.0
heated with ½ ounce brandy	.0
½ baked potato	10.5
topped with 2 tablespoons chived sour cream	1.0
1 cup cooked cauliflower, oven-heated	6.0
with 2 tablespoons grated Cheddar cheese	.2
total	18.4

MID-EVENING

2-egg omelette	.6
filled with 1 tablespoon grated Cheddar cheese	.1
cooked in 2 tablespoons butter	.2
total	.9

You've eaten six times in a single day and yet you've taken in a paltry 52.7 grams—well under your 60-gram limit. So you could, if you wished, add a quater of a cantaloupe melon to your dinner or luncheon menu (7 grams), or ½ cup of beets topped with 2 tablespoons of parsley sour cream (7 grams).

After just three weeks on her low-carbohydrate diet, Heather, who'd been wisely downing a multi-vitamin capsule every day too, shed those unflattering ten pounds. Ever since then she's remained loyal to this policy of low-carbohydrate intake, and despite the fact that she dines out constantly, Heather has remained a sleek 120 pounds.

THE FIVE-DAY DIET: A calorie counter. Personally, I find it fun to count calories. It makes me feel very efficient, and furthermore, it's proof positive that I'm not overeating. The secret here is what I like to call *The Art of Compensation.* You diet five days a week and then eat as you please on weekends, just so long as you don't exceed your weekly calorie limit.

How do you know how many calories you have to spend each day? This is a matter for you and your doctor to decide, based on your age, height, frame, and life-style. (If you're terribly active, as models are, you can consume more calories because you burn more calories than a less active person.)

Just for the sake of illustration, let's say you and your doctor decide you have a "bank" of 2,500 calories to spend each day. Ah, but spend only 1,200 of those calories for each of five days and presto! come Saturday morning you'll have spent only 6,000 calories instead of 12,500. That means you can s-p-l-u-r-g-e on the weekend and still the week's total won't add up to more than the grand total of 17,500 calories you're allowed. And if you think only 1,200 calories a day is meager fare, study this typical day's menu:

BREAKFAST	*Calories*
¼ cantaloupe	19
1 medium egg, poached	77
on 1 slice light rye toast	55
1 slice bacon, broiled	48
total	199

LUNCHEON	
5 canned artichoke hearts, chilled	25
with 2 tablespoons low-calorie French dressing	20
½ average chicken breast, roasted	110
½ cup banana whip pudding	85
½ glass skimmed milk	44
total	284

DINNER	
½ cup tomato juice	25
mixed with ½ sauerkraut juice	20
5 ounces red snapper, broiled	250
basted with ½ tablespoon lemon butter	50

33

DINNER (cont'd.)	Calories
1 cup shredded cabbage	24
with 2 tablespoons garlic vinegar	4
1 cup cooked spinach	45
1 cup diced cantaloupe	30
1 cup plain tea	0
total	448

A total of only 931 calories! So have another ½ cup of banana whip pudding (85 calories)—or better yet, skip it and really splurge on the weekend. Remember, you're permitted a week's total of 17,500 calories. So with this diet, it's the carrot-at-the-end-of-the-stick luring you on to a slimmer you.

A HIGH-PROTEIN DIET: Still another highly civilized and perfectly delicious way to lose weight. You eat all you want of certain high-protein foods. Follow the rules of this diet, and you don't even have to consider calories! And again, you're actually encouraged to eat six smaller meals each day rather than three bigger meals, the premise being that you'll feel less tempted to nibble between meals.

The approved high-protein foods . . .

Lean Meats—broiled, boiled, baked, or smoked. Butter, margarine, oil, or any kind of fat or grease are off limits both in the cooking and serving.

Chicken and Turkey—broiled, boiled, or roasted. With all skin removed. Again, no butter, margarine, oil, or fats.

Lean Fish, Seafood—broiled, boiled, or baked. And yes, you've guessed it—no butter, margarine, oil, or fats.

Eggs—even fried eggs just so long as they're made without using butter, margarine, oil, or fats (use a Teflon pan).

Cottage Cheese—in fact, any cheese that's made with skim milk rather than whole milk.

Dr. Irwin Maxwell Stillman, author of the best-selling *The Doctor's Quick Weight Loss Diet,* insisted on adding at least eight glasses of water daily to this high-protein diet, explaining that water was essential to wash away the residue of the body fat burned up via this diet. (And as far as I'm concerned, I drink a *minimum* of six to eight glasses of water a day, every day. I consider water a positive beauty essential.)

34

Norma Jean Dardin, one of the busiest black models posing today, lost almost a pound a day on a high-protein diet, going from a robust 140 pounds to a streamlined 123 pounds in well under one month. Norma Jean stands a statuesque 5'9" without heels, and while 140 pounds certainly didn't make her fat, "No model agency would touch me at that weight." It had been a proper figure while she was a Martha Graham dancer, but for a modeling career it was a drawback. So she concentrated on lamb chops and steaks for a week, then on the eighth day added halibut steak and chicken livers to her menu. Turning up her lovely nose at such things as butter, mayonnaise, sauces, salad dressings, and condiments, she concentrated instead on leafy greens, fruits, and cheeses made with skim milk. And *voila!* Norma Jean—top model—was born.

THE ADULT WEIGHT-REDUCING GUIDE: You don't find the Department of Health of the City of New York playing around with tricky diet names. It mails this diet to you in a regular envelope with an 8 cent stamp, for it's all of five skinny pages with such no-nonsense headings as "For Most Women and Small Men" and "For Most Men and Large Frame Women." The former get a daily 1,200-calorie menu plan, while the latter get a daily 1,600-calorie menu plan. Unlike the five-day diet, this is a seven-day-every-day diet with no weekend splurges, but if you suspect skullduggery (translation: sparrow feedings), just look at this typical 1,200-calorie menu plan:

Breakfast

Fruit—your choice of any one of the following: 1 large tangerine, 4 ounces unsweetened orange or grapefruit juice, 1 medium orange, ½ medium cantaloupe, ½ cup strawberries, 1 medium mango, ½ small papaya *(delicious!),* ½ medium grapefruit, 8 ounces tomato juice.

Protein Food—choose one: 2 ounces cottage or pot cheese, 2 ounces cooked or canned fish, 1 egg (no more than 4 eggs allowed a week).

Bread or Cereal—1 slice of enriched or whole grain bread *or* ¾ cup of ready-to-eat cereal *or* ½ cup of cooked cereal. (Skim milk with your cereal, of course.)

Coffee or Tea—*sans* milk and sugar.

Lunch

Protein Food—select one of the following: 2 ounces fish, poultry, or lean meat; 4 ounces cottage or pot cheese; 2 ounces hard cheese (no more than twice a week).

Bread—2 slices of enriched or whole grain bread.

Vegetables—raw or cooked, all you want except potato or substitute.

Fruit—any kind, 1 *small* serving, no sugar.

Coffee or Tea—*sans* milk and sugar.

Dinner

Protein Food—choose one: 4 ounces cooked lean meat, poultry, or fish.

Vegetables—raw or cooked, all you want, BUT make certain one has a high vitamin A content. Which are those? Any one of this list: broccoli, carrots, chicory, collards, dandelion greens, escarole, kale, mustard greens, pumpkin, spinach, swiss chard, turnip greens, watercress, and winter squash.

Potatoes? Yes, of course. Choose one (or a potato substitute) from this list: 1 medium potato, 1 small sweet potato or yam, ½ cup corn, 1 small ear corn, ½ cooked dry beans, peas, or lentils, ½ cup green peas, ½ cup lima beans, ½ cup cooked rice, spaghetti, macaroni, grits, or noodles.

Fruit—any kind so long as it's a small serving with no sugar.

Coffee or Tea—*sans* milk and sugar.

Exactly how effective is this diet plan? Well, it's the foundation upon which the Weight Watchers empire has been built. Need I say more?

GAYLORD HAUSER'S TEN-DAY DIET: Gaylord Hauser, dietitian, nutritionist, author, and all-around renaissance man in the twin fields of health and diet, began attracting attention back in the 1920s. Perhaps more than anyone else, he has made health foods sound glamorous and dieting sound like fun. I recently glimpsed him walking through the lobby of the Hotel St. Regis here in New York—a tall (6'3"), spectacularly trim (215 pounds) man who looks

36

as young today as he did when his book, *Look Younger, Live Longer,* zoomed to the top of the best-seller lists in 1950. His disciples (he refers to them affectionately as "my People") include some of the most glamorous women in the world, among them the perennially youthful Duchess of Windsor and Greta Garbo. He and his "People" are the most effective advertisements I can think of for his teachings.

Mr. Hauser's ten-day diet is another high-protein diet because, as he puts it, "First-class protein foods have a specific dynamic action and help to burn up fat." Since an all-protein diet, however, could create too much acidity, his diet contains plenty of fruits, vegetables, and milk. Vitamins A, B, C, D, and E are all here and accounted for in a diet that is chock-full of taste variety. But I think the big excitement for you is in the news that almost everyone who has faithfully followed this diet for ten days reports a loss of ten pounds. A POUND A DAY!

Picking a menu at random, here's one for the third day:

BREAKFAST

½ grapefruit

Clear coffee or café au lait (half coffee and half hot skim milk)

Fortify yourself with 1 fish liver oil capsule (vitamin A), 1 ascorbic acid tablet (vitamin C), 1 wheat germ capsule (vitamins B and E), plus mineral tablets containing calcium, phosphorus, iron, and iodine.

LUNCH

2 scrambled eggs
1 slice rye toast
Large sliced tomato
Clear beverage or fortified milk (special blend)

DINNER

Lean steak
Salad bowl
Fresh or broiled grapefruit
Fortified milk or demitasse

37

BEDTIME

Hot or cold fortified milk or glass of fat-free yogurt

If you're hungry between meals, Mr. Hauser urges you to nibble on celery or carrots, or fill up on a glass of fortified milk.

Fortified milk? I hear you say. Here is the Gaylord Hauser recipe for it and I heartily recommend it, even if you don't follow this ten-day diet. Keep a pitcher of it in your refrigerator and every time you drink a glass realize that you're getting protein value that, according to its creator, is equal to that of seven large steaks.

Pour into a blender the following ingredients: 1 pint of milk; 4 heaping tablespoons of brewer's yeast; 1 cup of powdered skim milk; 1 tablespoon or more of blackstrap molasses. When your blender has smoothed out this rich and healthy mixture, stir in another pint of milk. Stash it away in your fridge and drink, drink, DRINK!

ADAM AND EVE DIET: Apples are delicious low-calorie foods. Apples are also juicy sources of vitamins A and C. And furthermore, since they're so economical, they offer you a great way to fill up between meals. A good-sized, crunchy apple eaten slowly seems to normalize an otherwise greedy appetite. And who doesn't occasionally have an urge to eat between meals? I know I do, and so I keep apples around—both as food and decor. They look so attractive and cheery! Great hunks of Americana. There's always a silver bowl full of luscious red apples in our New York apartment, and in our home in the country I keep a wooden bowl brimming over with them—often as a table centerpiece.

Years ago the Swiss Fruit Association promoted an apple diet that became tremendously popular throughout that tiny country. Here's a menu from that diet:

BREAKFAST

large cup of café au lait
1 slice of slightly buttered rye bread

MID-MORNING

1 big juicy apple

38

LUNCHEON

large cup of clear broth
1 veal chop
Large serving red cabbage, cooked with apple
1 potato boiled with jacket
Green salad with oil and vinegar dressing

MID-AFTERNOON

1 big juicy apple

DINNER

2 hard-boiled eggs
1 slice of slightly buttered rye bread
Clear tea or café au lait

BEDTIME SNACK

1 big juicy apple

Perhaps that's a trifle too Spartan for your taste? Then improvise. Pick up a calorie counter at your supermarket or drugstore, stock up on apples (for variety's sake, try many different kinds), and go to it. AFTER a chat with your doctor, of course. Despite the old bromide that an apple a day keeps the doctor away, I urge you (AGAIN!) to consult your doctor before you begin any diet. This is the advice the head of any reputable model agency gives to any aspiring model who must shed poundage before she faces a camera. But perhaps no one does it with more authority than Wilhelmina Cooper, the former model who now heads up the agency bearing her name.

Statuesque Wilhelmina (5′ 10″) weighed a full-bodied 149 pounds when she started her modeling career. Her features were so exquisite and her physical proportions so harmonious that, despite her weight, fashion photographers used her, playing with lights and camera angles to camouflage her poundage. When she retired from modeling to open her agency in the late 1960s, Wilhelmina was a slim 125— "my best working weight." Sounds like a fantastic diet story, doesn't it? It was—finally.

Anxious to lose weight, Wilhelmina went on near starvation diets

39

(for example: for nearly two years, one bowl of soup a day, with a piece of melba toast in the morning so she wouldn't faint). Nevertheless, she somehow couldn't get below 139 pounds. Meanwhile, she was all but ruining her muscle tone by strapping herself into waist cinchers, girdles, and tight bras. Eventually her hair and nails began to show the effects of her scarecrow dieting. So she loaded up with vitamin pills. "I was piling them in," she recalls today. "I actually became allergic to certain vitamins. My complexion started breaking out." Finally, Wilhelmina sought out a doctor who listened to her story, sensibly came to the conclusion that it was impossible for a girl to starve herself and not lose weight, and discovered the cause—a tricky thyroid that at that point was practically down to zero. Once she began the proper treatments under the watchful eye of her doctor, Wilhelmina's weight went down as her thyroid went up. And the rest is history. She went on to become one of the most successful models ever, and today, like anyone who has learned the value of sensible eating, she remains wondrously slim and energetic—always in perfect control of her weight and able, in her own words, "to eat what and when I want."

I find the more you know about a subject, the more fascinating that subject becomes—and the more interesting you become. So read on and learn what our New York models know about the subject of staying sleek and glamorous.

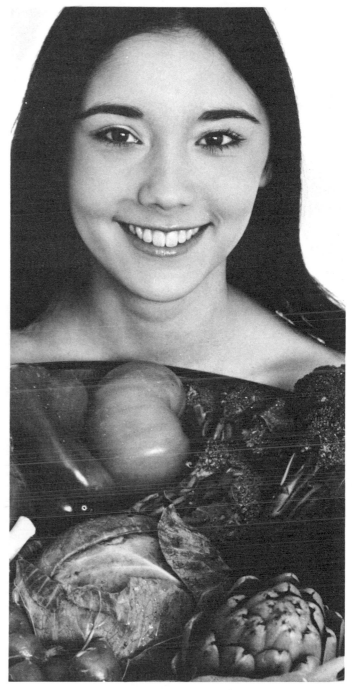

Aimee Liu loves fresh vegetables and knows that they are among the best sources of essential vitamins. Of course, there are lots of other luscious foods, too, that provide the important glamor vitamins.

CHAPTER · 4

Your Glamor
Vitamins

A successful model is always a healthy female, a veritable power-house of energy. On an average day she dashes all over the city, toting pounds of clothes, a makeup kit, and often a wig box. And there are more than a few of us who, despairing of traffic jams and taxicabs with "off-duty" signs, cover our rounds on a motor bike or a motorcycle. We're the seventies' models—the girls who, says Wilhemina, "look like girls but only a little more stretched out." But believe me, the waxen-looking models of the forties and fifties were—despite their hollow cheeks and heavy-lidded glamor—every bit as healthy and durable. They had to be. Stamina is one of the major requirements of the model business.

I suppose mine is a very practical viewpoint. I regard my body as a machine, and vitamins as its spark plugs. I believe that if you eat properly, you may never need to dip into a bottle of vitamin pills. But that is a matter for you and your doctor to decide. One thing is certain, however: vitamin pills must never serve as a substitute for natural foods. Your doctor will see to it that your diet supplies all the essential vitamins, but there's no time like now to learn which foods are bursting with rich vitamins.

Here are the glamor vitamins that help give models their smooth skins, shiny hair, sparkling eyes, strong nails and teeth . . . and *joie de vivre!*

VITAMIN A is what I call a skin food. And fortunately, it's simple to get your share of it in fresh yellow and green vegetables, and in that wonder meat—calf's liver. The following foods are extra rich sources of this happy vitamin:

Calf's liver	Squash
Spinach	Mustard greens
Carrots	Kale
Turnip greens	Pumpkin

42

Broccoli	Butter
Sweet potatoes	Eggs
Beet greens	Peaches
Dandelion greens	Green beans
Yellow corn	Asparagus
Apricots	Cantaloupe
Tomatoes	Eggplant

I take every opportunity to sneak Vitamin A into a menu, and I find carrots offer almost limitless opportunities. I chop them up into an otherwise green salad. I often make carrot cookies, using honey, egg, lemon juice—*delicious!* And here's my recipe for a Vitamin A-rich green bean salad:

> 2 pounds green beans, tipped
> Boiling salted water
> ⅔ cup olive oil
> 3 tablespoons cider vinegar
> 1 teaspoon salt
> ⅛ teaspoon freshly ground pepper
> 1½ teaspoons prepared mustard
> 2 medium onions, peeled and sliced thin
> ¼ cup minced parsley
> 2 teaspoons dried tarragon

Cook beans in the boiling salted water until they are tender but still crisp. While beans cook, mix remaining ingredients to make a dressing. Drain beans; place in a bowl. While they're still hot, add dressing and toss. Let stand at room temperature until serving time. Or cover and store in the refrigerator. Do not chill too long or the flavor will be lost. (6 servings)

VITAMIN B is a workhorse of a vitamin. There's a whole family of B vitamins that do splendid things for everything from your hair to your nervous system. Unfortunately, they aren't as plentiful in our foods as we might wish them to be. And so it's here that one turns to

43

the health food stores. For your guidance, the following foods are the very best sources of the B's:

Wheat germ	Fish
Brewer's yeast	Molasses
Yogurt	Loin of pork
Whole wheat breads	Kidneys
Whole wheat cereals	Nuts
Rice	Egg yolk
Soybeans	Lean smoked ham
Almonds	Dried skim milk
Sprouts	Roast leg of mutton

Yogurt has become so popular in the past decade that it's practically a staple item on most models' daily menu. In fact, this wonder food has become *so* popular that sometimes the dieter is rather indiscriminate and doesn't realize that some of the flavored yogurts are higher in calories than others—often climbing to a hefty near-300 calories versus the 118 calories found in an 8-ounce container of the plain yogurt put out by Dannon. Need I suggest you choose the plain rather than fancy while dieting?

Here let me give you the recipe for a fat-free yogurt that Gaylord Hauser provides in his marvelous book, *Look Younger, Live Longer*: "Add ½ cup powdered skim milk to 1 quart skim milk, and mix in an electric blender. Heat this mixture until it's good and hot, but don't let the milk boil. Into this hot but not boiling milk, stir 3 tablespoons ready-made yogurt. Pour this mixture into a milk bottle, or a double boiler, or any utensil, and place it in warm water, near the pilot light of your stove or near a radiator. Cover it with a shawl, much the same as you would raising dough for bread-making." In about five hours, you will have a quart of delicious fat-free yogurt.

VITAMIN C, the citrus vitamin, is my vitamin. I feel very possessive about it. Like most Floridians, I grew up with oranges and grapefruits practically within arm's reach. And I still can't think of a better way to begin a day than with a tall glass of orange juice. Happily for citrus addicts like me, vitamin C must be taken *every* day since it can't be stored in the body. Besides being available to you in fresh citrus fruits, this delectable vitamin is also found in the following foods:

Cauliflower	Red and green peppers
Spinach	Asparagus
Cabbage	Endive
Turnips	Peaches
Soybeans	Avocado
Lima beans, green	

Here are two of my favorite salad recipes using oranges, and both are chock-full of vitamin C:

Tossed Green Salad With Oranges, Avocados, and Onions

2 tablespoons mild cider vinegar
2 teaspoons grated orange rind
2 tablespoons fresh orange juice
1 tablespoon fresh lemon juice
¼ teaspoon salt
　 Freshly ground pepper to taste
¼ teaspoon dry mustard
½ cup salad oil (not olive oil)
2 large seedless oranges
½ avocado
1 medium Bermuda onion
1 large head romaine lettuce
½ medium head iceberg lettuce

Combine vinegar, orange rind and juice, lemon juice, salt, pepper, mustard, and salad oil in a jar with a tight lid; shake well. Pare and section oranges, being careful to remove all the white part. Peel avocado; halve, pit, and cut into pieces about the same size as the orange sections. Peel onion and slice thin; separate into rings. Combine orange sections, avocado, and onion rings in a bowl; pour dressing over mixture. Chill, covered, for several hours or overnight.

45

Trim salad greens and wash. Tear them into bite-size pieces. (Do not cut them because the leaves will darken.) Drain thoroughly in a colander, then on paper toweling; wrap in a kitchen towel and chill.

At serving time, place greens in a salad bowl. Add the chilled fruit-onion mixture with dressing; toss gently. Taste for seasoning and, if necessary, add a little more salt and pepper. (6 servings)

Orange and Onion Bowl

6 seedless oranges
1 medium-sweet red or white onion
¼ cup French dressing
¼ cup orange juice
   Boston lettuce

Pare oranges, removing all the white part; slice over a bowl to catch the juice. Slice onion thin; separate into rings. Make alternate layers of orange slices and onion rings. Mix French dressing and orange juice together and pour over oranges and onions. Cover and chill one hour.

At serving time, line a salad bowl with Boston lettuce. Drain orange-onion mixture; spoon over lettuce. (6 servings)

VITAMIN D is the sunshine vitamin, important for good bones and teeth. Before women became so keenly aware of the aging effects of too much direct sunlight on the skin, they often soaked up enough vitamin D via sunbathing to last all winter. Today there are many women who assiduously avoid exposure to the summer sun. I sunbathe but in moderation, and always protect against burning by lathering on a rich, moisturizing suntan lotion. I can't altogether avoid the sun, however, since I have a passion for golf, swimming, tennis, and sailing. Then, too, our New York apartment is a triplex penthouse, and who could resist exercising outdoors on a terrace that has such a breathtaking view of the East River! Furthermore, I grew up in Florida—and who ever heard of a Floridian seeking out the shady side of the street? But if you avoid the sun (models sometimes have to) and suspect you're not getting an adequate supply of vitamin D, think back to all those cod-liver oil capsules you probably

46

swallowed during childhood. They're a tried-and-true way to get your vitamin D *sans* sunshine. Fish-liver oil or halibut-liver oil capsules work just as well. In fact, whether or not you sunbathe during the summer months, I recommend you begin taking your vitamin D in capsule form at the very first gust of winter.

VITAMIN E is important for a strong heart, good muscle tone, and a healthy sex life. If you eat well, you get sufficient quantities of this vitamin. But most models I know take no chances and invest in a jar of Kretschmer Wheat Germ which, along with green lettuce and avocado, is one of the best sources of vitamin E. Since wheat germ contains not only vitamin E but the B vitamins and iron as well, I regard it as a king of nutritional insurance. Why, half a cup of it contains four times as much protein as an egg! Wheat germ makes a very tasty natural cereal, and you can also sprinkle it over your favorite fruit or salad. In fact, there are scores of low-calorie recipes using miraculous wheat germ, and you'll find some of the most delicious ones in Chapter 14.

Tanya Leveau has a very original way of filling up without filling out, while also getting a good amount of vitamin E. She buys a whole head of lettuce, shreds it, and then plumps the leaves into a frying pan just after she's finished whatever meat she's been preparing. She mixes the lettuce leaves with the dark meat juices, and then covers the pan and lets it steam lightly. She often devours a whole head of lettuce this way. It's a healthy, crunchy, deep-down satisfying way to pamper your taste buds and get your Vitamin E, without risking an extra pound.

VITAMIN K is needed for normal blood coagulation. If you eat a well-balanced diet, you won't miss out on your intake of this vitamin, which abounds in all the green leafy vegetables. Still, if you want to make doubly certain you're getting a fair share, dip a spoon into some fat-free yogurt—or mix up my favorite spinach salad and get a vitamin C bonus:

Spinach and Mushroom Salad

Wash ½ pound fresh young spinach in several changes of cold water. Cut off and discard the tough stems, dry the leaves thoroughly, and chill them. Arrange the

47

spinach leaves in a salad bowl and top them with 12 thinly sliced, firm mushrooms. Mix ½ cup French dressing with 2 teaspoons grated onion and 1 teaspoon Dijon-style mustard, pour it over the spinach, and toss. (4 servings)

One of the most scrumptious spinach and mushroom salads in all New York is served at P. J. Clarke's, the now almost legendary pub-restaurant on Third Avenue, where people such as famous model Veruschka, and Jackie and Aristotle Onassis, often sneak in for a late night snack. Next time you're nearby, make a point of visiting Clarke's and order their spinach and mushroom salad!

VITAMIN P, the least known vitamin, is valuable to normal blood pressure. Its best sources are citrus fruits and green peppers, both of which you're certain to use no matter which diet you and your doctor decide on.

As I said before, dieting is an adventure in eating!

Yolande Catharina Flesch adores cantaloupe, a rich source of Vitamin C that does beautiful things for your skin. Furthermore, 1/2 pound of this scrumptious and very filling fruit adds up to only 34 calories!

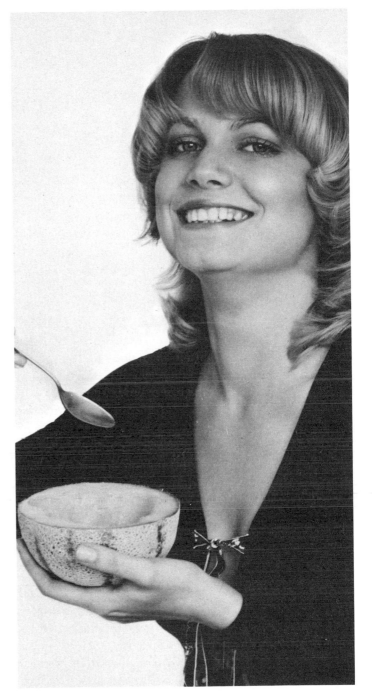

CHAPTER · 5

For Smooth,
Healthy Skin

The purpose of the various encounter groups that have mushroomed throughout the United States is to help you realize your "Human Potential." Well, I have a way to help you recognize your "Beauty Potential": wipe off all makeup; shampoo your hair and towel dry; then, take a good look into your mirror and see what you *really* look like.

Is your complexion—when free of powder, blusher, and whatever else you use—smooth and fresh-looking? Is your hair shiny and bouncy? The answer should be YES to both questions, but if that isn't your answer, don't despair. Proper diet is the first step toward healthy, young-looking skin and hair, and happily you are about to start your own very special diet. Couple these sensible eating habits you're about to learn with knowledgeable care of your skin and hair, and you'll be on your way to attaining what is the very basis of a model's success. For skin and hair comprise a woman's presence—give her her aura of femininity. Without a lovely complexion and equally lovely hair, an aspiring model has little chance of success. On the other hand, many a relatively plain girl who had these two important attributes has become, with the magic of makeup, a *beauty*.

So, here are some plain facts for unplain girls.

Beautiful Skin Foods:

Protein: Cheese, eggs, fish, poultry, meats, dried beans.
Vitamin A: Eggs, as well as all those lovely and leafy yellow and green vegetables listed under this vitamin in Chapter 4.
Vitamin B: Whole wheat bread, cereals, and all those healthful foods listed under this vitamin in Chapter 4. (Skimp on this vitamin, and dry skin will be your "reward.")

HOW TO REMOVE MAKEUP: No matter how late it is or how very tired I am, I never retire without knowing I have deep-down clean skin. Here's my nightly ritual, recommended for *normal* and *dry* skins.

With my fingertips, I apply baby oil all over my face and neck. Then, with tissues I remove all makeup and oil residue via what I call my *mini-facial*—sweeping up-and-out motions. Next, I apply a second coating of oil in exactly the same way, repeating my mini-facial with clean tissues. (I insist on using white tissues for they clearly tell me when my skin is deep-down clean.)

Perhaps you don't really feel clean without soap and water. In that case, use soap and water after applying the oil once. Instead of tissues, use a face cloth, and work with an up-and -out motion.

Follow the cleansing with an application of a liquid moisturizer to your face and neck.

POSTSCRIPT FOR DRY SKINS: Avoid a regular thick washcloth and use your fingertips instead (you could use a thin, very soft cloth). Dry skin can't take too much friction. Choose a bland soap and *warm* water: hot water is drying. And so is steam heat, so I suggest you buy a humidifier for your bedroom, or at least that you counteract the drying effects of steam heat by having a dish of water in the bedroom while you sleep. When possible, of course, sleep with an open window.

HOW TO REMOVE MAKEUP FROM AN OILY SKIN: Remove makeup with a nongreasy cleansing cream. Next, go to work with a medicated soap, *hot* water, and a scruffy washcloth that will help stimulate circulation. Rinse with cold water and apply an astringent (witch hazel will do fine) to close your pores. I also recommend that once a week you take advantage of the detergent action of cleansing grains, paying very special attention to the oiliest areas of your face.

BEDTIME GLAMOR: Personally I detest going to bed with an oily looking skin (and I think most husbands feel the same way about their wives!) So I get rid of that "salad" look by dampening a face cloth with lukewarm water and, using my mini-facial motion, gently patting the cloth all over my skin, removing every smidgen of oily residue. Then, with my fingertips I apply a liquid moisturizer to my face and neck. Final touch: a little liquid rouge on cheeks and lips for a fresh, natural-looking glow. I feel clean because my skin *is* clean, but I don't look like a comic strip wife. I feel glamorous—and I think that is important.

FACIAL MASKS: These are temporary skin rejuvenators; they stimulate surface circulation and tighten pores. Some masks are ideal for all skin types, while others are specialists. But no matter what kind of mask you choose, it *must* be applied to a deep-down clean skin. So remember to cleanse your skin according to your skin type *before* applying your mask.

Egg Mask for Rough-Textured Skin: Crack an egg and beat the white until it's a froth. Add a tablespoon of strained honey, plus a half teaspoon of lemon juice (fresh or bottled). Mix thoroughly. With your fingertips apply the mask all over your face and neck. Leave it on for no less than 20 and no more than 30 minutes. Remove with a towel dipped in lukewarm water. Immediately dab on skin freshener. NOT recommended for dry skins.

Buttermilk Mask for Oily Skins Only: Mix powdered buttermilk with water as directed on the package. Since you must not allow the mask near your eyes, you will have to lie down when applying it. Protect your eyes with cotton pads soaked in cold water or witch hazel. When applying the mask, pay special attention to your oily skin areas. Leave the mask on for 15 to 20 minutes, then remove it with a towel dipped in lukewarm water. Apply a lubricating cream. Remove the creamy residue with tissues, and pat on an application of a skin freshener.

Oatmeal Mask for Oily Skins Only: Mix a paste of dry oatmeal and warm water. Put it on your face and neck, and let it dry. Then remove at once with clear, cold water. Follow with an application of skin freshener.

Honey-and-Egg Mask for Dry Skins Only: Beat together one egg yolk and a tablespoon of strained honey. With your fingertips apply the mixture all over your face and neck. Leave on for 15 to 20 minutes. Remove with a towel dipped in lukewarm water.

52

Honey Mask for All Skin Types: Using one tablespoon of strained honey at room temperature, with your fingertips apply the honey all over your face and neck. This is naturally very sticky and you must be very gentle as you apply it to the delicate skin around your eyes. The trick is to actually massage the honey into your skin, by pressing your fingers on your skin and then pulling them away—a not unpleasant sensation! Leave the mask on for 15 minutes. Then remove it by pressing a towel dipped in warm water all over your face and neck. Immediately follow up with a towel dipped in cold water.

If your skin is *oily,* use a skin freshener.

If your skin is *dry* or *normal,* use a lubricating cream.

Note: Some people urge you to steam your face before applying any facial mask. That is, cleanse, then steam. I disagree. I believe intense heat applied directly to the face is too drying. So, unless you have an extremely oily skin, I maintain that the cleansing ritual I've described is quite enough preparation for applying your facial mask.

Oleda and her sister, Frances Petty, know that proper diet is essential for healthy, bouncing hair. (By the way, there is a nine-year difference between the two sisters—Oleda being the older.)

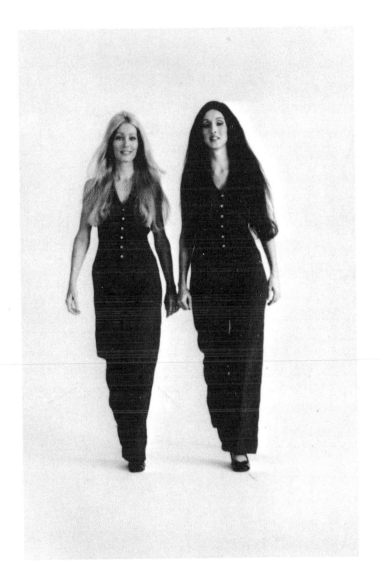

CHAPTER · 6

For Shiny, Healthy Hair

My hair is waist-length and I color it. Nature darkened my naturally blonde hair when I was still a child, but since I still felt like a blonde—fancied I had a blonde personality—I soon decided to color my hair. I've been coloring my hair for more than a dozen years, yet it has so much shine that often when I do a television commercial, the hair stylist has to powder my hair down. So you see, there is absolutely no reason for any woman to have dull hair, unless of course she's a victim of overbleaching or an "overcooked" permanent.

Beautiful hair is healthy hair and healthy hair is clean hair. So let's approach this subject in exactly that order.

Foods for Healthy Hair

Protein: Cheese, eggs, fish, poultry, meats, dried beans.
Vitamin A: The beautifier for both skin and hair! So
    check under this superb vitamin in Chapter 4.
Vitamin B: Ditto.

How to Shampoo for Best Results

There's no magic to shampooing, only a little shower of common sense.

Always begin by brushing your hair to take out any tangles and remove any loose dust that may have settled on your hair. Next, massage your scalp with your fingertips. Don't pinch your scalp. Simply spread your fingers and keeping them stiff, rotate and gently lift your scalp.

IF YOUR HAIR IS DRY, use a pure castile-soap shampoo. It contains the nourishing oils your hair type requires. Rinse your hair

56

four or five times—removing all soap film to achieve a high shine. Towel dry, then follow with a cream rinse or conditioner to give your hair glamorous highlights and the body that dry hair too often lacks.

IF YOUR HAIR IS OILY, use a soap-based shampoo that will give you a truly bubbly lather. Rinse, rinse, and rinse again—thorough rinsing is positively vital. Towel dry and use a cream rinse, then treat your hair to a beer rinse—it will give your hair a bouncy manageability. Stale beer is preferable and by stale I mean a can or bottle of beer that's been opened for at least several hours. A day is better. If you don't have stale beer, follow this routine and you'll have a reasonable facsimile: Open a fresh can or bottle and heat it in a pan. Allow it to cool and then use it. A half can or bottle is the amount to use. Put the remaining half (*covered*) back into your refrigerator. You'll be able to keep it for weeks, provided there's no sign of mildew. Pour the beer slowly through your hair and do *not* rinse out—just set.

Remember always to comb very gently while setting, since hair is weakest and most liable to break when it's wet.

Beauty Aids From Your Supermarket

Your supermarket is a positive treasure chest of beauty aids for your hair. They may be in traditionally plain wrappers or in their natural state, but, believe me, they hold the key to glamorous hair.

OLIVE OIL, for instance, does wonders for dry hair when used as a conditioner before shampooing. Here's how to use it: Pour warm olive oil into a cup and apply it directly to your scalp. Then wrap a hot towel turban-fashion around your head. Just as soon as the towel cools, put a fresh hot one on. Repeat this procedure for 20 or 30 minutes. Unfurl your towel and massage the oil into your hair. Next, apply your last fresh hot towel and keep it on for a full *60 minutes*. To remove all traces of oil, I suggest you shampoo a minimum of three times with lots and lots of rinsing.

57

VINEGAR, the cider variety, is a marvelous rinse for brunettes, giving their hair dazzling highlights. White vinegar does the same for blondes. Here's the recipe: To three glasses of lukewarm water add four tablespoons of vinegar. Massage this tangy mixture into your hair and then remove the vinegar scent via lots of clear, cool water.

TEA is a redhead's best rinse. Brew according to directions on the package. Strain and mix with a pint of water. Pour the mixture through your hair and then rinse with clear, cool water.

LEMONS are, I think, the favorite rinse of most "natural" blondes. I rather suspect their appeal has something to do with the blondeness of the lemon and its provocative scent—not to overlook the gleam and sheen it adds to all shades of blonde hair.

Mix the strained juice of two lemons with two glasses of lukewarm water. Pour the mixture through your hair. If your hair is dry, rinse with clear, cool water; but if it isn't, I suggest you skip the rinse and, if possible, let your hair dry in the sunshine. The combination of lemon juice and sunshine inevitably adds highlights even to blonde hair.

EGGS are practically sacred to all sorts of purists who consider the egg one of nature's architectural masterpieces. Eggs are nearly sacred to crafty models, too, who eat them for their vitamin content and use them externally for hair and complexion beauty.

The egg shampoo is a perfectly glorious shampoo for all types of hair: Crack two or three eggs into a bowl, separating the white from the yolk. Whip the whites until they froth. Then, after plopping the egg yolks into a cup, add a tablespoon of water and blend until you have a creamy mix. Now mix froth and cream together for a *frothy cream* that all but begs for a color camera. Wet your hair with warm water, then with your fingertips apply some of the frothy cream to your scalp. And I mean *really* apply it, massaging gently until it's all worked in. Rinse in cool water and apply more of the frothy cream. Repeat the application and rinsing until your egg mix is all used up. Be sure to rinse thoroughly—*squeaky clean*—and towel dry.

58

Treatments for Problem Hair

We Give Great Haircuts, Inc. is the name of a fantastically chic emporium located on Manhattan's East Side. Catering to women only, it's tucked in the basement of an apartment building, and is one of a string of colorful shops and boutiques that have sprung up on East 53rd Street. Jacques Lawlor is the owner of We Give Great Haircuts, Inc. and besides doing what the shop's name promises, handsome Jacques and his young assistants work to bring problem hair back to health. American-born, luxuriously bearded Jacques studied with Vidal Sassoon, and since he's been his own boss, he has evolved a series of common-sense treatments using organic shampoos in conjunction with natural foods and, in a few instances, even strained baby food. Many models credit Jacques Lawlor with keeping their hair in prime condition. He was generous enough to confide some of his secrets to me, and here they are:

Treatment for damaged hair:
1. Shampoo with an organically grown shampoo that is available at any really well-stocked health food store. Apply the liquid shampoo to hair while it's dry. If you prefer to wet your hair first, Jacques suggests that you use no more than an ounce of water. (He believes water forms a wall between hair and shampoo and thus makes it more difficult for the shampoo to work.)
2. Rinse thoroughly. Leave your hair wet.
3. Then, a mixture consisting of one tablespoon of lemon juice (natural or the bottled kind) and two ounces of strained liver baby food should be applied directly to your hair and scalp.
4. Wrap your head in a hot towel for approximately 15 minutes—or sit under a dryer for 15 minutes with a plastic bag covering your hair.
5. Rinse thoroughly.

Treatment for not-so-damaged hair (excessively dry hair, split ends, or simply hair not as pliable or shiny as it should be):

59

1. Apply approximately two serving spoons of mayonnaise to your hair after shampooing. Jacques says the vinegar in mayonnaise separates the hair and lets light in—and light reflecting through hair is what makes it shine.
2. Wrap your head in a hot towel for 15 to 25 minutes, or sit under a dryer with a plastic bag covering your hair.
3. Give your hair *two* more shampoos, rinsing thoroughly.

Treatment for dandruff:
1. With a brush (a round brush, Jacques specifies, with bristles approximately 1/4 inch apart), rough up your scalp to loosen dandruff flakes.
2. In a regular-sized coffee cup prepare the following mixture: one inch of warm water; 30 aspirin tablets dissolved in the water and mixed with your finger; ½ tablespoon baking soda, and mixed with your finger (be prepared: this will foam and run over the sides of the cup).
3. Shampoo with an organically-grown shampoo.
4. Do *not* rinse, but add mixture directly to hair, working it into your hair and scalp with your fingertips. Leave combination of shampoo and mixture on for 15 minutes.
5. Rinse.
6. With a fine tooth comb, gently work over your scalp to remove any remaining dandruff flakes.
7. Repeat this treatment every day for one week.

Treatment for oily hair:
1. Add one teaspoon baking soda to the amount of organic shampoo you will use (approximately ¼ cup for short hair, ½ cup for long hair). Soda absorbs oil like a sponge, says Jacques.

OR

2. Powder on pure talcum powder and then use organic shampoo. A pure talcum, containing no perfume, also removes excess oil from hair.
3. If your hair is oily, eliminate nuts, butter, chocolate, and fried foods from your diet.

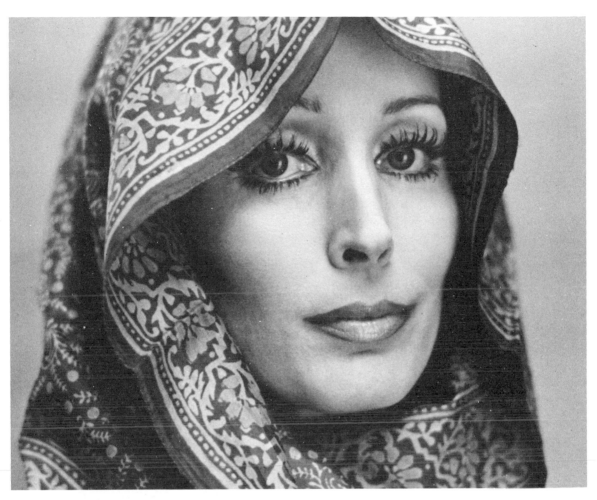

For sparkling and clear eyes, Oleda believes in eye drops and eye exercises, as well as vitamins A and B. *(Photo: Steve Ladner)*

CHAPTER · 7

There are fashions in makeup just as there are in clothes. One season it may be red-red lips and nails, and eye makeup as colorful as a mosaic. Then the next season a pale look is in, and even false eyelashes may be peeled off and tucked away for safekeeping; then everything is *au naturel!*

Happily, however, some things remain constant, such as sparkling, strong eyes. They're never out of style. Even if they're shaded by false lashes and glamorized with scrumptious shades of shadow, eyes must be healthy and expressive in order to be alluring. All of which dictates that the whites of the eyes be snowflake white, and the irises and pupils sparkle with vitality. Even when utterly devoid of makeup, eyes like that are beautiful to see. Makeup only adds to their natural beauty, and makeup, no matter how artfully applied, can never camouflage eyes that are tired and lack luster.

If eyes are to be sparkling and strong, they must be "fed," just as hair and skin must be "fed."

THE EYE BOOSTER VITAMINS: Vitamin A does wonders not only for your skin but for your eyes, too. Those fresh yellow and green vegetables work magic by helping the tear ducts secrete the natural moisture which, in turn, helps give our eyes their natural sparkle.

And then there's vitamin B, that workhorse of a vitamin that seems never to stop doing good for us. As we've already noted, there's a whole family of B vitamins, and for eyes it's B_2, also known as riboflavin. That's the super-duper vitamin, since it not only helps beautify the skin and eyes, but also builds and maintains body tissue by helping our cells use oxygen.

The best sources of vitamin B_2? Here's the list:

Eggs	Lean meats
Enriched bread	Calf's liver (also top of the list
Enriched cereals	of vitamin A foods)
Leafy green vegetables (here's	Dried yeast
where vitamins A and B_2	Milk
join forces)	

64

The Natural Vitamin Foundation recommends 0.6 milligrams of vitamin B_2 per 1,000 calories in your diet, and never less than 1.2 milligrams daily.

The National Dairy Council recommends two or more glasses of milk a day for adults, and four or more for teen-agers. But if milk doesn't appeal to you, bear in mind that cheese, ice cream, and other milk-made foods can supply at least part of your milk requirement.

CLEAN, CLEAN EYES: After all, how can you expect your eyes to sparkle if they're not sparkling clean? Eye drops are as much a part of a model's clean-up ritual as brushing her teeth. I urge you to put drops into your eyes before retiring and again first thing in the morning. And yes, invest in a pocket-sized plastic bottle of your favorite eye drops and carry it in your handbag. Clean, clean eyes have always been a beauty essential, but never more than today when we live in a smog-glutted environment.

ISOMETRICS FOR YOUR EYES: When I was a teen-ager, I read a beauty story that detailed Ginger Rogers' recipe for captivating orbs. A very important part of it was eye exercise. Now, quite frankly, it's just possible that that beauty tip was born in the fertile imagination of a Hollywood press agent. But I do know that, even today, the vivacious Miss Rogers' sapphire blue eyes have a gem-like sparkle. I like to believe that it's due to her eye exercises. At any rate, Ginger Rogers inspired me to begin eye exercises, which I've never stopped and never will stop doing.

I regard exercises for the eyes to be as essential as exercises for the figure and face, particularly today when so much of our time is spent looking at a television screen. Too much of our looking is confined to short distances, so we must take time out to "stretch" our eye muscles to work beyond the six to eight feet between us and the video screen, the eight to ten inches between us and our magazine, book, or newspaper. I'm often shocked to see just how many Americans wear eyeglasses. Watch a television camera pan over a studio audience and see the lights reflecting off that sea of eyeglasses! Certainly if you must wear glasses, wear them, for to strain your eyes is sheer lunacy (and there are scads of attractively designed frames to choose from). But I rather suspect that many Americans take to spectacles because of lazy eye muscles, just as many women take to girdles because of lazy body muscles.

65

A dynamic woman lives in an apartment only a block from ours. Her name is Elizabeth Gilfillan and she teaches facial isometrics. Miss G. is about ninety, yet her skin is still smooth and lovely. *And* this remarkable woman doesn't wear eyeglasses. She's a firm believer in eye exercises. So let's say that both Ginger Rogers and Elizabeth Gilfillan are the twin inspirations for the following eye exercises that I do every day of my life—often twice a day:

1. This one is my eye warm-up exercise. Slowly roll your eyes clear around, starting at the far left, then up over the top, down to the far right, along the bottom and back to the far left. Repeat for a series of six eye rolls, and then do another six, this time starting at the far right and moving counterclockwise.
2. Looking straight ahead, blink both eyes quickly to the count of ten.
3. Sit straight and look straight ahead. Now, look up and out to the left as far as you can *without turning your head.* Count 1-2-3. Next shift your eyes so that you're looking up and out to the right as far as you can without turning your head. Do this six times.
4. Still sitting straight and looking straight ahead, raise eyes toward the ceiling slowly without tipping your head back (or wrinkling your forehead). Now, quickly drop your eyes down and, without tipping your head down (or tucking in your chin), try to see your feet. Neither will be possible of course, but the attempt will be a marvelous exercise for fatigued eye muscles.
5. Sit or stand by a window that permits you a long-distance view, and *stare* ahead just as far as your eyes will see. Oh, what a fabulous feeling! It will be as though your eye muscles were stretching, and actually it also seems to smooth your brow in the process. (So many of those unhappy looking frown lines between the brows come from squinting in close quarters.)
6. Complete your eye isometrics with this tried-and-true eye relaxer: Cup a hand over each eye, gently pressing the heel of each palm onto your cheekbones so that

you see nothing but inky black. Once you've totally blacked out all light concentrate on that blackness for a slow count of ten.

Follow your eye isometrics with two drops of eyewash, then pat a little moisturizer or oil on the delicate skin under and beside each eye, and I guarantee you'll be ready to see eye to eye with this cockeyed world of ours!

Lots of dairy products and good dental care help give Eleanor Poole her beautiful strong white teeth.

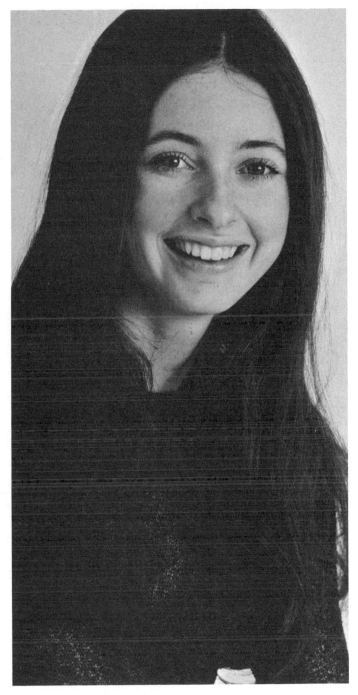

CHAPTER · 8

For Strong,
Sexy Teeth

The sexy smile, the goal of every model and every woman, is a healthy smile—shining teeth with good color and firm, strong gums.

Diet and exercise concepts also apply to the care of teeth and gums. Modern dentistry offers insight into the prevention of decay and gum disease (the most universal of ailments), and stresses that care by the patient himself is essential—the foods you eat and don't eat, and your methods of oral cleansing. A dentist friend of mine, Harold Schwartz, who teaches at New York University Dental School, told me about new research data that definitely pinpoint ways to prevent deterioration of teeth and gums. Models conscious of health and beauty factors seek out the best and newest methods in dentistry.

Research points to dental "plaque" as the culprit. Plaque is an adhesive-like substance that sticks to the surface of the teeth and gums and is filled with millions of micro-organisms carrying bacteria that cause diseases. Initially plaque has to be professionally removed, but it is the patient's responsibility to keep it from coming back. A three-point home care program is usually part of the treatment to do away with plaque.

1. Daily use of nonwaxed dental floss in-between the teeth is most important.
2. Washing thoroughly with a Water Pik.
3. Brushing with a soft brush, having rounded nylon bristles. Brush *across* the teeth, not in the old up-and-down direction.

Studies carried out at New York University, Columbia University, University of Texas, and at the National Institute of Health, confirm these new methods. Ask your own dentist. If he has not yet read the latest literature, prod him! He will be delighted to have an ally in the care of your teeth.

70

And what about diet for the smile of beauty? Is it true that candy, cake, white bread, and gum are the harbingers of those evil refined sugars and carbohydrates? It is! Sucrose is the problem substance, and it is found in those delicious foods that you shouldn't be eating for other reasons, too. Fructose, found in natural fruits, is the answer to your craving for a sweet dessert. But if you must, one rich dessert a day is better than nibbling sweets constantly.

The American Foundation for Medical-Dental Science, a nonprofit corporation operating in Beverly Hills (lots of sexy smiles out there!), also urges a full quart of milk daily and not less than one egg per day.

What to Eat to Get It

The best sources of calcium (so essential to healthy teeth and bones, as well as a serene nervous system) are:

> Milk
> Cheese, especially
>   cheddar cheese
> Ice cream
> Turnip and mustard greens
> Collards and kale

The best sources of phosphorus (for building and maintaining good bones and teeth) are:

> Milk (again!)
> Egg yolks
> Fish
> Meat
> Cheese
> Whole cereals
> Peas and beans

Now feast your eyes and smack your lips over these nutritious

71

recipes which the Foundation says will satisfy your sweet tooth while protecting teeth and gums.

Fruit and Nut Pastry Roll

2 eggs
2 teaspoons baking powder
Generous ⅛ pound butter
2 pounds whole grain flour
(if desired ½ cup of soy bean flour may be mixed with whole grain flour)
1 whole ground lemon, including rind and juice

Complete mixture should be moistened to cookie dough texture with approximately 3/4 cup hot tea.

Filling: Grind together 3/4 cup each of nuts, white raisins, prunes, dates (other dried fruits may be added or interchanged with these mixtures according to choice). Add grated rind of one lemon; 2 tablespoons of honey may be added, if desired.

Roll dough flat to about 3/8 inch thickness, spread filling mixture, roll, sprinkle top lightly with mixture of cinnamon and sugar, slice and bake in hot oven (350°F.) for approximately 30 to 45 minutes.

Fruit Square

Grind together ½ pound dried apricots, ½ pound dried prunes, 1 cup walnuts, 1 apple seeded and peeled, 1 cup dates, 3 tablespoons preserved ginger. Shape into squares 1 X 2 inches.

Baked Custard

Beat 4 eggs with rotary or electric beater, add ¼ teaspoon salt, 3 tablespoons honey. Continue beating and gradually adding 2¼ cups hot, but not boiled, milk and 1 teaspoon vanilla. Beat together well. Place in baking dish, sprinkle top with nutmeg, set in pan of hot water and bake in moderate oven (325–350°F.) for about 45 minutes. (Serves 6)

Custard Sauce

Beat the yolks of three eggs slightly, add ½ teaspoon salt and 2 tablespoons honey. Stir constantly and add 2 cups scalded milk. Cook in double boiler until mixture thickens. Just before serving stir in either ½ teaspoon vanilla or ½ teaspoon rum. May be served hot or cold.

What Not to Eat (in any substantial quantity):

Candy	Jelly
Cookies	White sugar
Pies	Brown sugar
Cakes	Packaged (ready-to-eat)
Doughnuts	cereals (the Foundation
White bread	argues for the whole grain
White flour	cereals that require cooking)
Soft drinks	

Your dentist can perform simple chemical tests to find out your caries (tooth decay) susceptibility. He will be happy to discuss your diet habits and can then intelligently advise you about an individual health care program. The amount of caries is related to form and frequency of ingestion. One example: caramels and toffees will cause greater incidence of decay than sweetened bread or chocolate.

Research studies show a remarkable and immediate rise in dental caries when some people switch from caramels, sour balls, et al. Get a pacifier! But give up smoking! It stains the teeth and causes mouth odors, among other known horrors.

Fluorides in drinking water is a *fait accompli* in most communities, and long-standing research proves that it really works. The more ways you use fluorides, the less susceptible to decay you will be, especially if you are under thirty. Use a fluoride dentifrice and mouth wash. Have your dentist apply fluorides locally twice a year when he cleans your teeth. If caries are really your special problem— you cannot have a sexy, appealing smile with decaying teeth—the dentist may recommend use of a fluoride Gel. He will make a plastic mouth-guard to help you apply it yourself each night. This method can reduce caries up to 85 percent. Also ask your dentist about new

73

sealants that can be applied to your teeth to shield them from harmful bacteria.

SPECIAL NOTE: If you have children, see to it that they make their first visit to the dentist at the age of three. This is considered the ideal time to lay the groundwork for good communication between child and dentist. And do bear in mind how important it is to take proper care of baby teeth if strong second teeth are to grow. You're advised by the experts to help the child brush. It's a proven medical fact that children don't begin to coordinate well until about their seventh year.

Preserving natural teeth in a state of good health is the easiest and best way to a beautiful and sexy smile. The old-fashioned straight-edged super-white grin has gone the way of all artificial concepts of beauty. Slight individual imperfections in tooth position can be interesting and attractive, as long as the teeth are healthy.

Although modern dentistry offers specialized means to perfection in tooth appearance, the best way to prevent dental breakdown is through proper diet and daily home care procedures, under the guidance of your dentist.

If necessary, the dentist can move teeth or he can restore and replace decayed or missing teeth with artistic, functional jackets, crowns, and bridges. And tell him you want sexy teeth that are designed for your shaped face, size, age, and coloring. The contemporary dentist considers these factors essential to his patient's psychological health, as well as a natural appearance. For the person with tooth problems, modern dentistry offers new painless methods and creative restorations.

Sexy teeth with a natural look for today's world is the message of healthy, beautiful models.

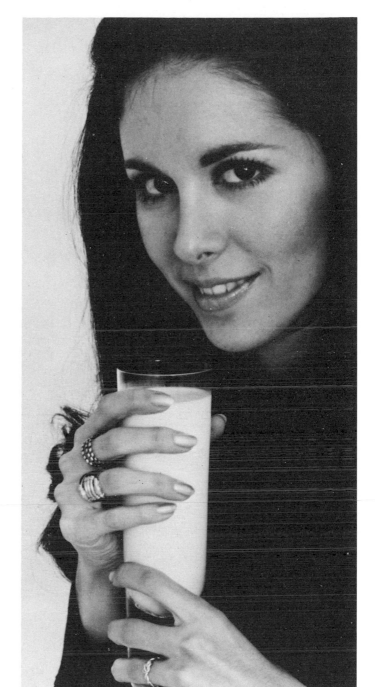

Dana Carroll believes in
drinking milk every day for
pretty hands and strong nails.

CHAPTER · 9

For Soft,
Alluring Hands

Hands up! And if you're caught red-handed, shame on you. There's absolutely no excuse today for hands that are anything less than soft and smooth. But if yours are rough and red, follow this simple home remedy for one week and you're sure to get good results:

1. Soak both hands in *warm* water for just a few minutes.
2. Pat dry and coat both hands with petroleum jelly. This will lubricate and soothe them. Tissue off the excess.
3. Each day—several times a day—apply a creamy hand lotion. (Pour some into a small plastic bottle and keep it in your handbag.)
4. At bedtime, rub in an extra-rich cream and slip on a pair of thin cotton gloves; then keep them on all the while you sleep.

THE DELUXE HOME MANICURE: Heather Hazell has very elegant hands, with an incomparably creamy color, and strong, long, and very beautiful nails. Furthermore, Heather is her own favorite manicurist. Here is her weekly hand care ritual:

Before her manicure, Heather rubs in a rich cuticle cream and then pushes down the cuticles with an orange stick that has a small, soft eraser on the tip. (You can simply cushion the blunt end of an ordinary orange stick with cotton.)

She files down and rounds off the tops of her nails, never touching the sides. This, she says, is the secret of their great strength—letting them grow straight at the sides. "I never get broken nails!" she boasts.

She gives her nails *two* base coats on top, and then puts *two* under the *tips* of her nails. That way her nails are fortified on both sides. Next are applied *two* coats of color, then a top coat over and under her nails. Midweek, or about every three days, she puts another base coat over and under, just to keep her nails strong. Three times a week she uses a nail cream she describes as "very rich, very gloppy," massaging it into her cuticles to keep them soft and pushed back.

FINGERNAIL FACTS: Pat Barrie is one of the busiest of all hand models. She's also a very thorough type, and so she's accumulated a stockpile of fingernail facts. She calls it trivia, but I call it fascinating and I think you will, too:

> Children's nails grow faster than adults'.
> Nails grow faster in the summer than in the winter (so does hair).
> Nails grow 70 percent faster on fingers than on toes.
> The little finger and thumb nails grow more slowly than the other nails.
> If, as a child, you had measles or mumps your nails will not grow at the normal rate.
> Undernourishment (lack of protein and vitamins A, B, C, and D in your diet) causes the nails to be extremely slow in growth rate.
> Nails, unlike hair, do not breathe and need all the protection you can give them.

FINGERNAIL FOODS: For strong, no-chip nails essential to beautiful hands.

Protein: Cheese, eggs, fish, poultry, meats, dried beans.

Calcium: Milk, powdered skim milk, cheese, buttermilk, yogurt.

Iron: Raisins, liver, molasses, whole wheat, apricots, oysters.

Pat Barrie supplements her diet with gelatine, which she considers absolutely essential for really strong fingernails. So once every three days Pat adds water to a packet of Knox's flavored gelatine, stirs quickly, and drinks it down. If you have weak nails, she advises you to follow this routine faithfully *every* day.

And happily, there are now many slimming dishes that include Knox Gelatine as an integral part of the recipe. Here are some that Pat recommends and that I've tried and found perfectly delicious.

77

RECIPES USING KNOX GELATINE

Gelatine dishes may be made in molds, bowls, or individual dishes. The individual dishes or bowls are simplest for family service; for the company table, molded dishes look most handsome. If you are concerned about how to unmold, be assured—it is most simple. Dip the mold into a bowl of warm (not hot) water to the depth of its contents. Run a small sharp paring knife around the rim. Top the mold with a serving plate, invert, and shake gently. If the contents don't slip out readily, repeat the procedure.

Curried Confetti Ring

2	envelopes Knox Unflavored Gelatine
3½	cups cold chicken stock, divided
1	tablespoon curry powder
1	teaspoon salt
⅛	teaspoon pepper
1	cup mayonnaise
2½	tablespoons minced onion
1	cup chopped celery
¼	cup chopped pimiento
4	hard-cooked eggs, coarsely chopped

Sprinkle gelatine over 1 cup cold chicken stock in saucepan. Add curry powder. Place over moderate heat, stirring constantly, until gelatine is dissolved, about 4 to 5 minutes. Remove from heat. Add remaining 2½ cups chicken stock, salt, pepper and mayonnaise; beat with rotary beater until smooth. Add onion. Chill, stirring occasionally until mixture is consistency of unbeaten egg white. Fold in celery, pimiento and hard-cooked eggs. Turn into 6-cup ring mold. Chill until firm.

Chicken Salad

½	cup mayonnaise
1	tablespoon minced onion

1 tablespoon lemon juice
½ teaspoon salt
⅛ teaspoon pepper
3 cups diced cooked chicken
1 cup diced celery
1 cup seedless white grapes
½ cup slivered toasted almonds
  Curried confetti ring

Combine mayonnaise, onion, lemon juice, salt and pepper. Add chicken, celery, grapes and all but 1 tablespoon almonds. Mix lightly. To serve, unmold curry ring. Fill center of ring with chicken salad. Sprinkle with reserved almonds and garnish with greens. (8 servings)

Bean Pole Salad

2 envelopes Knox Unflavored Gelatine
2½ cups cold water, divided
1 tablespoon onion flakes
½ cup tarragon vinegar
½ cup sugar or equivalent
  nonnutritive sweetener
1 teaspoon salt
½ cup chopped pimiento
1 can (1 pound) whole green beans, drained
1 can (4 ounces) sliced mushrooms, drained

Sprinkle gelatine over ½ cup cold water in saucepan; stir in onion flakes, place over low heat; stir constantly until gelatine dissolves, about three minutes. Stir in remaining 2 cups water, vinegar, sugar or nonnutritive sweetener, and salt. Chill until mixture is consistency of unbeaten egg white. Fold in pimiento, beans and mushrooms. Turn into a five-cup mold. Chill until firm. Unmold. (6 servings), 96 calories per serving with sugar; 30 calories with nonnutritive sweetener.

Asparagus Aspic

1 envelope Knox Unflavored Gelatine
1½ cups cold water, divided
3 tablespoons white vinegar
1 teaspoon salt
4 teaspoons sugar
⅛ teaspoon Tabasco
1 cup cut-up cooked
   asparagus spears
1 tablespoon chopped parsley
1 tablespoon finely chopped celery
¼ cup diced pimiento

Sprinkle gelatine over ½ cup cold water in saucepan. Place over low heat and stir until gelatine dissolves, about three minutes. Stir in vinegar, salt, sugar, Tabasco and remaining 1 cup water. Chill until mixture is consistency of unbeaten egg white. Fold in remaining ingredients. Turn into a three-cup mold. Chill until firm. Unmold to serve. (4 servings), 23 calories per serving.

Slim Line Snow

1 envelope Knox Unflavored Gelatine
1¼ cups cold water, divided
¾ cup sugar or equivalent
   nonnutritive sweetener
¼ cup lime juice
2 teaspoons grated lime rind
2 unbeaten egg whites
   Green food coloring

Sprinkle gelatine over ½ cup cold water in saucepan. Place over low heat; stir constantly until gelatine dissolves, about three minutes. Remove from heat. Stir in sugar or nonnutritive sweetener, remaining ¾ cup water, lime juice, and rind. Chill until slightly thicker than consistency of unbeaten egg white. Add unbeaten egg whites and a few drops food coloring; beat with rotary beater or electric mixer until mixture is fluffy and begins to hold its shape. Turn into a six-cup mold or bowl; chill until firm. Unmold. (6 servings), 113 calories per serving with sugar, 13 calories with nonnutritive sweetener.

80

Applesauce Whip

1   envelope Knox Unflavored Gelatine
1   cup cold water, divided
    Nonnutritive sweetener, equivalent to
        ⅓ cup sugar
1   teaspoon grated lemon rind
2   tablespoons lemon juice
2   cups unsweetened applesauce

Sprinkle gelatine over ½ cup cold water in saucepan. Place over low heat; stir constantly until gelatine dissolves, two or three minutes. Remove from heat; stir in remaining water, sweetener, lemon rind and juice, and applesauce. Chill, stirring occasionally, until mixture mounds slightly when dropped from spoon. Beat with rotary or electric beater until light and fluffy. Turn into six dessert dishes. (6 servings)

EXERCISES FOR ALLURING HANDS: Tanya Leveau is always in demand as a hand model, too. In fact, in her very first television commercial, her hands were all viewers saw of this little beauty. Now, please don't ask me why Oriental women have such lovely, expressive hands. I don't know. Ask Tanya and she confides that she took piano and fife lessons when she was a child. She suggests that perhaps it was all that five-finger exercise. I like to think that it's because Oriental dance and pantomime both concentrate on hand movements. Whatever the reason, Tanya's hands are breathtakingly lovely, and here are some very simple hand exercises she recommends "to keep hands flexible and fingers well defined."

1. Place both hands flat on your lap, palms down. Now, pretend your hands are fans that are about to open—slowly. This means spreading your fingers in slow motion. Spread them to the every extreme . . . hold for the count of 5 . . . and then snap each "fan" shut. Repeat six times.
2. Clench a fist. Hold it tightly (the way a baby does when he's gotten hold of something), and then fling your hand open with all fingers spread. Repeat six times.

3. Pick up a rubber ball and *squeeze* your fingers into it as though you were trying to puncture it. Repeat six times.

Models, like actresses, must know how to use their hands to express a mood. A tweedy suit designed for long walks in the country, for example, asks for a very different hand gesture than does, say, a velvet evening gown. Both Tanya and Pat use their hands so eloquently that they add immeasurably to the mood of whatever it is they're modeling for, whether a shampoo or a kicky swimsuit. And one beauty tip they both recommend is to keep hands up when in repose. Not only do they look more graceful that way, but it also makes the veins in the hands less noticeable (and we all have veins in our hands!).

HAND-ME-DOWNS: Before we leave the subject of hands, let me pass on a few of my own beauty tips:

Never soak your nails in oil, as that will soften them—contrary to what some beauty editors claim.

Never rub your fingertips through tinted or dyed hair.

For a hand beauty massage: Use a hand cream or a face cream and massage it into your skin, starting at your fingertips and stroking up over the backs of your hands and past your wrists. (I know scads of models who are wild about the new beauty products made from natural oils of fresh fruits and vegetables—yummy sounding things like an ambrosial peach body moisturizer, pink strawberry cleansing cream and a green avocado hand cream. I've tried the hand cream and love it.)

Special color chart for hands: If your skin is sallow, the nail polish colors you'll find most flattering are in the beige-pink range.

Anti-polish? Buff your nails to bring out their natural gloss. Rub buffing polish around your nails with a chamois-covered buffer. A dozen or so buffings in one direction will do the trick.

82

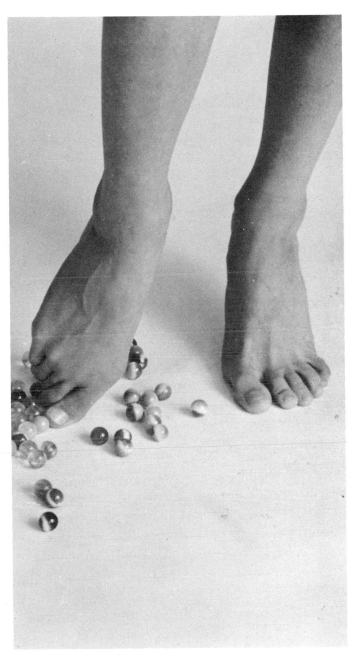

Picking up marbles with your toes is one way of exercising many of the foot muscles.

CHAPTER·10

For Pretty,
Pretty Feet

I believe our feet are without a doubt the most neglected, most abused part of our anatomy. Until summertime. Ah, then we go to work pampering those woebegone appendages, hoping that the tell-tale signs of neglect can be coaxed away with a crash program of foot baths, pumice stone, and waves of creams and lotions. Sometimes it works. And sometimes it doesn't. And when it doesn't, those unsightly calluses, bumps, and blemishes (I won't even mention *corns!*) strip a femme of her glamor even if she's fortified with a ravishing bikini and a silky suntan. When it works, we are grateful; but do we sensibly break the anti-foot cycle neglect in winter, pampering in summer? Rarely. Well, I say it's high time we stopped this nonsense. Your feet should be every bit as lovely and seductive as your hands, and today—with fashion dictating so much exposure of epidermis—they'd *better be.*

Besides being the hardest working part of your entire body, your feet contain one quarter of all the bones in your body—26 in total. So naturally it's vital that your diet contain those foods that make for good bones.

FOODS FOR PRETTY, PRETTY FEET: Vitamins C and D are essential. Check back to Chapter 4 and you'll find a list of the goodies that are richest sources of both these vitamins. Since sunshine is a prime source of vitamin D, you should, of course, seize every opportunity to get your feet sun, air, and freedom.

Calcium is the mineral for good bones and teeth. Best sources are:

> Milk
> Cheese, especially
>   cheddar cheese
> Ice cream
> Turnip and mustard greens
> Collards and kale

EXERCISES FOR PRETTY, PRETTY FEET: Judy Brown has the sleekest, prettiest feet any girl could hope for. See a closeup of feet *au naturel* or in a pair of revealing sandals on television or in a magazine advertisement, and nine times out of ten those sexy feet belong to Judy. So it's not surprising that she's a veritable walking encyclopedia about feet. And, according to Judy, to improve the muscle tone of your feet there is nothing more effective than the following exercises:

1. Rise on tiptoe twenty times each day. And after the first week, she suggests you add to this exercise by walking about on tiptoes. Frontward. Backward. Sideways. Walking on tiptoes this way is not only good exercise for your feet, but it will also tighten your tummy and buttocks.
2. Sit on the edge of your bed and cross your legs. Hook your handbag over the ankle of your top leg and do six push-ups. That is, raise and lower your foot by circling your toes up and down, causing your handbag to rise and fall slowly. Do six push ups with one leg, then six with the other. This exercise not only tones up the muscles of your feet but exercises your ankles, too. After all, satiny smooth, lithe feet deserve trim ankles, don't they?
3. Toss a handful of marbles on your carpet and try to pick them up with your toes.
4. Plunk the bulkiest telephone directory you can find down on your carpet. Next, drape a hand towel over it. Now, draw up a straight-back chair, sit down on it, and plant your two feet firmly on the phone book with toes over the edge. Practice trying to pluck the towel off with your toes.

BEAUTY TREATMENT FOR PRETTY, PRETTY FEET: To keep her feet looking and feeling satiny smooth, Judy Brown takes to her tub with a pumice stone twice a week. In the warm tub water, she uses it to smooth the backs of her heels and the bottoms of her feet.

A pedicure is a twice-a-month affair for Judy. And here's the way she advises you to do yours to achieve the most glamorous results:

85

1. Soak your feet in warm, soapy water.
2. Towel dry and then clip nails almost straight across.
3. File your toenails smooth.
4. Push back cuticles with a cotton-wrapped orange stick.
5. Massage your feet with a camphored cream, really kneading it into the skin.
6. Rub half a lemon over each foot. (Judy claims it helps keep skin exquisitely white and fine-pored.)
7. Puff with cooling talcum powder. In fact, Judy urges daily talcuming, maintaining it's as necessary to foot beauty as brushing is to hair beauty.
8. Apply polish to nails.

STILL MORE TIPS ON FOOT CARE (culled from 101 models):

For swollen feet: A foot bath containing Epsom salts.

For perspiring feet: Splash on witch hazel that's been cooled in your refrigerator.

To avoid calluses: Soak for ten minutes in a solution of fluffy tannic acid powder and warm water. This combination "tans" the skin of your feet, creating a kind of shield against calluses.

For tired feet: Alternating hot and cold foot baths.

For healthy, straight-boned feet: Dance every chance you get. Walk barefoot every chance you get—indoors on carpeting, outdoors on grass or sandy beach. The combination of bare feet *and* sun *and* fresh air is the ideal beauty prescription.

For proper-fitting shoes: Buy yours in late afternoon, when your feet tend to be swollen and are most sensitive to fit.

Should you need further incentive to convince you that the time has come for you to give your feet the attention they deserve, let me pass on a nugget of common sense a famous cosmetic surgeon once delivered in a speech: *"Women are from their feet up!"*

Need I say more?

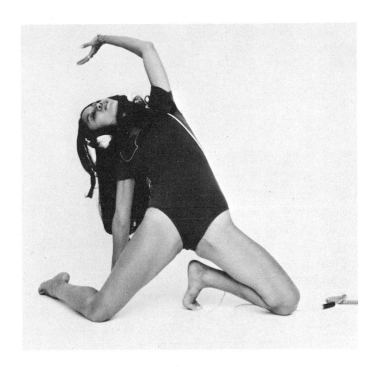

EXERCISING NEEDN'T BE A BORE

Tanya, an individualist in every way, dons a pair of earphones and dances her way through exercise sessions—fashioning her movements to suit her own mood and the mood of the music. Chris Palmer creates her own exercises, too. She stretches each part of the body as much as possible—and looks beautiful doing it.

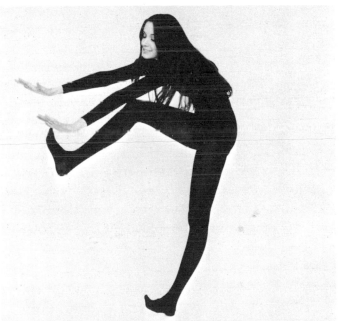

CHAPTER · 11

Our "Wouldn't-Live-Without-'Em" Exercises

Regular exercise—not haphazard hit-or-miss exercise—is what counts. There are still far too many women who sit and spread all winter long and then, at the first sight of a bud or bird, suddenly become figure-conscious and plunge headlong into a crash diet *plus* a crash exercise program designed to slim them down before they put away their winter clothes. Crash exercise programs are as silly and often as dangerous as crash diets!

Exercise should be as much a part of your daily routine as brushing your teeth. It needn't be strenuous. In fact, those old huff 'n puff exercises are terribly outdated. Simple exercises done for, say, ten minutes each day are enough to keep you slim and supple. An exercise program started now, and coupled with your diet, will bring your slender new figure to the fore that much sooner.

It's very important that you start now if you're going to avoid the disappointment that so many dieters face when they reach their ideal weight and discover that slim as they are they aren't fit. Remember that excess weight forces muscles to strain to support that poundage. When the extra pounds melt away, the body sags unless those muscles have been firmed via exercise. We've all seen slender women whose figures sag. And frankly, I find that perhaps even *more* unattractive than the overweight figure, for it's such an out-and-out sign of sheer laziness.

As Dr. Jean Mayer, Professor of Nutrition at Harvard University, has said: "Combating overweight by diet alone is like fighting with one hand behind your back. Exercise is the other fist that enables us to deal the knockout blow."

The following exercises will help you do exactly that. They're simple—and simply marvelous! They'll firm and tone your body, so that when you've attained your ideal weight, your figure will be youthfully supple.

If you have a particular figure problem, concentrate extra attention on those exercises designed for your problem area.

For the Waistline

1. Pretend you're a glider, and extend your arms out to the sides at shoulder level. Stand straight with legs about eighteen inches apart. Now, tip your "wings" as far to the left as you can—taking care to keep both knees from bending or your heels from rising off the floor. Bend so that you can feel the pull at your right side. Straighten up, and then bend to the right. Tip your "wings" 6 times on each side.

2. You're still a glider with both wings extended. But now instead of dipping those wings, you're going to attempt to turn, once again without bending your knees or lifting your feet off the floor. Back and legs must remain perfectly straight. Now, swing from the waist just as far as you can to the right. And like a good pilot, turn your head to see where that right arm is going. *Where* is it going? Just as far back as it can go without moving your feet. Return to starting position. Then, swing from the waist just as far as you can to the left. Do this exercise 6 times in each direction.

    My mother has done these two exercises for as many years as I can remember, and she has a scrumptious 28-inch waistline at 60-plus.

3. With feet still about 18 inches apart, back and knees straight, raise both arms straight up over your head. Slowly, *very* slowly, bend back both hands at the wrists until palms face the ceiling. Then, slowly s-t-r-e-t-c-h as though you felt you could touch the ceiling. When you've stretched as far as you can go without rising off the floor, hold to the count of 6. Relax and bring your arms down to your sides. Do 8 repetitions.

89

For the Stomach

1. Stand straight, with feet together and hands at your sides. Inhale slowly as you very slowly tighten the tummy muscles. Keep tightening until you feel as though you've practically got them pushing up against your spinal column. Hold that position to the count of 10. It's a tougher exercise than it may seem, and so I suggest you do it only once but repeat it several times during the course of the day. The nice thing about this exercise is you can do it anytime, anywhere.

2. This is my favorite. Onto the floor you go, lying flat on your back with both arms down at your sides. Lift both legs up at the same time, keeping your knees straight. Inhale as you lift legs perpendicular to your hips. Now, exhale as you slowly lower both legs *almost* to the floor—but not quite, stopping about 6 inches above the floor. Hold to the count of 3 and then raise again, inhaling as your legs start rising. This exercise really tugs at those tummy muscles, so 3 repetitions will be enough at the start. Work up to an eventual 6.

   There's a modified version of this exercise that I often do when I'm at my writing desk or in private just sitting and watching television. Shimmy to the edge of your chair, extend both legs straight out in front and raise them until both legs are at a level with your chair seat. Hold to the count of 3 and then lower slowly *almost* to the floor, stopping about 6 inches above the floor, and hold to the count of 3.

3. Lie on the floor on your back, arms at your side, palms down. Now, slowly raise both arms overhead until the backs of your hands are resting on the floor. The idea is to keep your feet flat on the floor all this time, and the way to do that is to let your knees relax slightly. So there you are—knees slightly bent, arms back with palms facing the ceiling. Now, try to lift your hips off the floor, while pulling in those tummy muscles. Relax and repeat. This, too, is a tough exercise, so do 3 repetitions to start and eventually work up to 6.

4. Lie on the floor on your back, arms at your side, palms down. Slowly raise your head and shoulders from the floor as you extend your left arm straight ahead in perfect synchronization with your right leg as it rises slowly from the floor. Continue this movement until the fingers of your left hand touch your right foot in mid-air. Hold to the count of 2, and return to your starting position on the floor. Repeat, this time touching your left foot with the fingers of your right hand. This is a positive *must* for the new mother whose tummy muscles may still be a bit flabby.

5. Lie on the floor on your back, arms straight back and palms facing the ceiling. Sit up quickly, swinging your arms forward and jackknifing your knees to your chest all in one motion. (*Important*: keep your toes pointed, elbows stiff.) Return to starting position on the floor. This one's a "toughie." Start with 2 repetitions, and gradually work up to 6.

For the Bosom

1. Standing, lock your hands before you with your elbows bent. Fingers entwined, press your palms together. *Press*—as though you were trying to press them together permanently. Repeat 6 times.

2. Standing, feet slightly apart, with a book (or a can of food) in each hand, raise your arms sideward to shoulder level, and start drawing circles in the air—small tight circles getting larger and larger, then smaller and tighter. Be certain to keep circle sizes of both arms uniform.

3. Sitting straight on the edge of a chair, take a book (or can) in each hand. Raise arms to shoulder level, bending elbows until elbows are at shoulder level, palms turned toward face. Now, very deliberately raise both arms overhead, bringing them together so that books actually touch—both arms extended straight up. Slowly return to shoulder level, elbows bent. Relax and repeat a total of 6 times.

For the Legs

These are all Judy Brown exercises, for the best reason I know: she has the loveliest legs I've ever seen!

1. Rise up on your toes and start walking! This is a truly superb leg exercise—and something of a derriere slimmer, too. Walk straight ahead, then sideways, then in reverse. Toe around for two to three minutes.

2. Plop a hard cover book on the floor. Stand with the balls of your feet on it. Now bounce on your heels very gingerly. Repeat this calf slimmer 10 times.

3. Lie on the floor on your back with knees bent. Start to pedal slowly. To keep your balance, *and* your hips on the floor, place your hands at your waist. Count 25 to 30 kicks. A great thigh slimmer!

4. Another one for the *thighs.* Sit on the floor grass-hopper style: soles of your feet facing each other and so close to your body that you're practically sitting on them. (Be slow and deliberate getting into this position, unless you're already very supple.) Now, cross your hands in prayer position around your toes. Hold that position, and *slowly* bend from the waist until your forehead touches your feet. Hold to the count of 3. (Mmmmm . . . feel that delicious tug on the thigh muscles?) Return to the starting position—slowly. This too, is difficult, so I suggest you start off with only 2 repetitions and slowly build to 6.

5. Sitting, cross your legs. Point the toes of your top leg toward the ceiling and then down toward the floor. Do this 25 times. Recross your legs and do the exercise 25 times with your other foot.

For the Hips

1. Lie on your left side resting on your left elbow, legs together. Bend your right leg at the knee with your toes pointed to the left knee. Now, raise your right leg straight up, then bend and lower again to the starting

92

position. Remember to inhale as you raise your leg and exhale as you lower it. Do this 6 times with each leg.

2. Stay on the floor! Here's another hip-slimmer. This time kneel on your knees and bend forward with both palms flat on the floor. Next, extend your left leg to the side, keeping your knee stiff and toes pointed. Now, raise and lower that left leg. Make it a *fast* movement. Do 12 with the left leg, then twelve with the right. Work up to 20 times with each leg.

For the Derriere

1. *This* is one exercise that practically every model I know does with gusto! Start in a sitting position on the floor. Put both legs straight in front of you, knees together. Raise the right knee, taking care to keep your right foot flat on the floor. Next, lower your right leg as you raise the left knee and start "walking," shifting weight from one buttock to the other as you move. It goes like this: lower right leg, raise left knee; lower left leg, raise right knee. Move ahead as far as you can, and then shift to reverse until you return to the spot where you started. Cover the length of the room.

   This, by the way, was the exercise Norma Jean Dardin did to make the transition from being a Martha Graham dancer to becoming a top model.

2. Stand tall, and lean both hands on the back of a chair or couch—in other words, a chair or couch high enough to *enable* you to stand tall. Without bending the torso one bit, kick your left leg back as high as you can without tipping over. (*Important*: keep your toes pointed, knees stiff.) Once you've discovered your limit, return to the starting position and proceed—in *staccato* fashion—to do 8 repetitions. Repeat 8 times with the right leg.

3. And here's *my* derriere firmer-upper. It's a sly one—so sly, in fact, that it can't be photographed. Far too sub-

tle, but *you* will feel it work. I do it when riding in an elevator, or standing at a corner waiting for a traffic light to change, or in a department store waiting for the saleslady to get around to me. Here's what you do: "Dig" both feet into the ground, seeming to grasp it with your toes as you nip in the buttocks. Hold it to the count of 5 and relax. Repeat. Nobody'll know you're doing it but you!

For the Upper Arm

1. This is so simple and so very effective! And since I'm such a great advocate of *preventive* measures, I advise you to start doing it even if you are dewy young and your upper arms are marvelously slim and firm. And if they *aren't,* don't waste another moment. Simply stand tall with both arms at your side, make two fists, and slowly extend your arms backwards and up as far as they can go. Hold that position to the count of 6 and bring the arms down to the starting position. *Stay* fisted and repeat 6 times.

    Marianna Heiser swears by this one, and I know some models do it with small cans of fruit juice in each hand (feeling it makes for even a stronger grip than a fist does). I leave that up to you, but remember the g-r-i-p is important.

    Tanya Leveau is slim as a reed, her lithe body as expressive as her lovely hands. And she intends to keep it that way. In the privacy of her apartment Tanya rarely sits in a chair or on a sofa. She perches—often like a glamorous grasshopper—when she's watching television.

    Tanya is an individualist in every way, even when it comes to exercising. Rather than follow a set exercise plan, she improvises. She slips into leotards, turns on her hi-fi, and *lets go.* She stretches. She rolls. She kicks.

She undulates. She lets her body respond to the music as it *feels* the music. And how Tanya feels one day may not be the way she'll feel the next day. But as you can see from the photograph of Tanya "responding," these unorthodox exercises do wonders for her figure.

Oleda's mother, Thelma Freeman, is past 60 and has done facial and neck exercises for years. She believes it's never too early to start.

CHAPTER · 12

*Exercises
for Your Face
and Neck, Too*

Facial isometrics are enormously popular today, but my mother—and my mother's mother—were doing them long before they had such a "scientific" name. I recall my mother, always a tremendously energetic lady, boasting that she exercised "from head to toe." She still does. Every day. And so should you.

Men have practiced facial isometrics for generations, whether or not they've realized it. Just watch a man when he's shaving and you'll see what I mean. The neck stretches. The chin line slides from side to side. The bottom lip protrudes. He may not regard those contortions as facial exercises, but they are—and very good ones, too. You'll discover that several of the following facial exercises bear a striking resemblance to the limbering up a man gives his face and neck every time he shaves.

For a Younger Looking Neckline

1. Open the collar of your dress or housecoat or whatever you're wearing, so that neck is completely exposed. Then, stare into a mirror with the most deadpan look you can muster. *Really* expressionless. Now, think of something amusing—downright silly, if you wish—but refuse to permit yourself to smile. Oh, let the corners of your mouth start to curve up ever so slightly at the edges but then force them to stop—to freeze in that position. Just the whisper of a smile, and then *tighten* so that it goes no further. Hold for the slow count of six. Do you see what happens? As you fight

98

your smile, the muscles on each side of your face flex clear down to your breastbone. Repeat this exercise 10 times.

2. Every time I do this one, I can't help but imagine the late Maurice Chevalier craning his neck to look at the top of the Empire State Building. A giddy thought, but I suggest you bear it in mind—it will help you do the exercise properly.

    Start by putting on a Chevalier mouth. You know, protrude the bottom lip as far as you can. Got it? Hold it, and now tip your head back until you're staring up at the ceiling—or the top of the Empire State where King Kong once stood clutching Fay Wray in his paw. Now pretend you can't see the top (too cloudy) and so you're disappointed. What do you do? You pull the corners of your mouth out toward the sides. Feel those neck muscles tighten? Clear down to the breastbone again. Hold that position for a slow count of 1-2-3. Maintain the Chevalier pout with the corners out toward the sides, but return your head to the starting position. Do the exercise again, tilting your head back and facing the top of the Empire State Building. In all, tilt the head 5 times.

For a Firmer Chin and Neck

Sit with your knees pulled up to your chest. Make certain you are sitting perfectly straight. Now, stretch your neck, taking care that you don't raise your shoulders in the process. Next, tilt your head down in front, then slowly lift your chin up and drop your head back. Keep going back as far as you can, and while you're doing this open and shut your mouth slowly. When you've gone back as far as you can, bring your head forward again, leading with your chin. Repeat 5 times. This is an absolutely smashing exercise, and it's really not fair to claim its magic for chin and neck alone; it actually improves your posture, too—and your posture, with which your neck is intimately involved, holds one secret of youth.

For a Firm Chin Line

1. Lower your chin onto your chest. Now, as you begin to cry a very slow and very exaggerated MEOW! slowly raise your head until, by the time you've finished your cat cry, you're looking up at the ceiling. At this point you'll find that you've lifted not only your head but your chin line as well. In fact, your lower lip should be protruding in the Maurice Chevalier style again. Hold to the slow count of 1-2-3. Now unlock the protruding lower lip as you very slowly lower your head to its normal position, but try to maintain the lifted chin line for as long as you can. (My mother boasts she can hold it for a good 20 to 25 minutes!) Repeat this exercise a minimum of 3 times.
2. Roll your head slowly, deliberately, stretching your neck as you make a complete circle going clockwise. Next, make a complete circle counterclockwise. Do both circles 6 times.
3. Stick out your tongue as far as you can, and then try to curl the tip until it touches the tip of your nose.

For Smooth Skin Under the Eyes

Place the fingertips of your 3 middle fingers very, very gently on the skin directly below the bottom lid of each eye. *Don't* press but simply rest them there without pressure of any kind all during this exercise. Now, very slowly raise the lower lid upward until the eye is practically shut. Open and repeat for a total of 5 repetitions. IMPORTANT: Don't raise your eyebrows, squint, or wrinkle your forehead while doing this exercise. All the motion must come from the lower eyelids only.

For Youthfully Rounded Cheeks

Place your index finger vertically over the very center of your mouth. Press gently and hold. Now, try to blow your finger away.

100

You can't, of course, but the more you try the more your cheeks puff out. Repeat 10 times, each time holding the puff to the slow count of 3.

For a Luscious, Youthful Mouth

Say *church* ever so slowly, as if you were Liza Doolittle and your very own Professor Higgins was there at your elbow trying to get you to enunciate clearly—C-H-U-R-C-H! Again. C-H-U-R-C-H! Each time exaggerate the word to the point that the tips of your upper lip practically collide with the tip of your nose. Repeat 6 times.

101

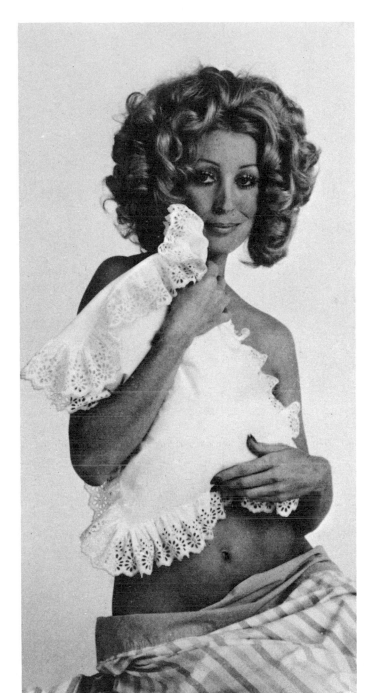

Sleeping in the nude with a
baby pillow is Oleda's way of
getting more beauty sleep.

CHAPTER · 13

Beauty Sleep
and How to Get It

I'm always amused at Hollywood's depiction of a model's life. If a working model were to follow the play-'til-the-wee-hours-of-the-morning life style that filmmakers imagine she does, she'd be out of the business within a month!

We sleep an average of eight hours a night. A *minimum* of seven. For we must never look anything less than fresh and rested. And neither should you, even if the only photograph you anticipate is a snapshot taken in your backyard. Sleep is rejuvenating. Sleep is blissful. And it's particularly essential while you're dieting, when it's so important that you always feel refreshed and cheerful.

Of course getting into bed at a sensible hour is no guarantee of a good night's sleep. I suggest you begin at the beginning—with the proper mattress—not one that sags under your body weight, but one firm enough yet flexible enough to give where it should and to support where it should.

I'm such a fanatic on the subject of sleep, I wangled an invitation to visit the factory of the Simmons Company, makers of the justly famous Beautyrest mattress. There I picked up the following tips on how to select a mattress.

Press down with the heel of your hand on one coil of the mattress. The coils on either side should remain firm, indicating that this mattress has a construction that permits each coil to act individually—quite like the keys of a piano. A mattress with these individual springs will give you the levelized body support you need. Mattresses with wired-together springs, on the other hand, sag down together, causing a valley. Result: haphazard support.

Lie down and *really* test the mattress. Try it out like you do a new pair of shoes. Spring action isn't enough, you see. It must be long enough and wide enough to guarantee you the stretch-out comfort you need.

Sleeping in the old-time feather bed is like being enfolded in a giant marshmallow: comfy, but deadly for the body. Don't be afraid of a

104

firm mattress. If you have a psychological need for something soft, why not make it a fluffy blanket?

According to my informant at the Simmons Company, ten to fifteen years is the usual life span of a good mattress. So if yours is an old-timer, it's high time you thought of getting a new one. A *firm* one.

Perhaps you've caught the marvelous 1933 film, *Dinner at Eight,* on television? If you have, then I know you must recall Jean Harlow's satin bed replete with white satin sheets and huge pillows drenched with lace. Ugh!

Satin sheets might be sensuous delights—I can't say because I've never had the urge to sample them. (I think I'd giggle as I slipped between them.) But I know I have no tolerance for huge pillows with or without lace. In fact, I don't even have tolerance for the ordinary-sized bed pillows, because they get in my way. I want to control my pillow, not vice versa. So I prefer a *baby* pillow. That's right, a *baby* pillow. I buy mine in the infants' shop at a local department store, and by now the saleslady knows me and has stopped asking, "How old is the baby?" My baby pillow is a sweet 10 inches wide, 3 inches high, and has a baby pillowcase.

The first time my mother-in-law saw my baby pillow, she laughed. But when her visit was over the following week, she packed one in her travel bag. I didn't have to sell her on the idea of switching; she sold herself by trying my pillow one night. The next morning she found that, for the first time in years, her "early morning face" looked and felt much smoother. Why? Because a baby pillow plumps down to practically nothing. An ordinary-sized pillow, however, fights back, and during the night your face crunches down into it—and loses the battle. Next morning you see the "battle scars": those temporary lines and wrinkles around the eyes and below the cheeks. Oh, they do iron out soon enough, but as you grow older you'll find they look deeper and last longer.

Another thing, a plump pillow props your head to a level that practically invites a double chin. A baby pillow, on the other hand, actually supports the neck muscles. More and more women I know have switched to baby pillows. Actress and beauty columnist Arlene Dahl, for instance, has slept on a baby pillow for years—she even travels with it. Get one of your own. It's a neck-saver.

105

I also believe that some nightwear fabrics are restful, while others are naggers. The naggers are the pesky fabrics that slip and bind and interfere with your rest. Long ago I substituted cotton for the slippery silks, satins, rayons, and nylon. And I grade loose-fitting pajamas much higher than a figure-hugging nightie. Should wearing loose-fitting pj's strike you as being too much of the Girl Scout, then dare to sleep nude. Your body needs air. And you'll be amazed at how much more refreshed you'll feel the next morning.

If falling into an easy, natural sleep is a problem for you, don't reach for a sleeping pill. Instead hie yourself off to the kitchen and prepare something that will contribute to your relaxation. Here are two drinks that I recommend as sleep inducers:

A glass of hot grapefruit juice sweetened with a teaspoon of strained honey; or a glass of hot water with two teaspoons of lemon juice and a teaspoon of honey.

Sweet dreams!

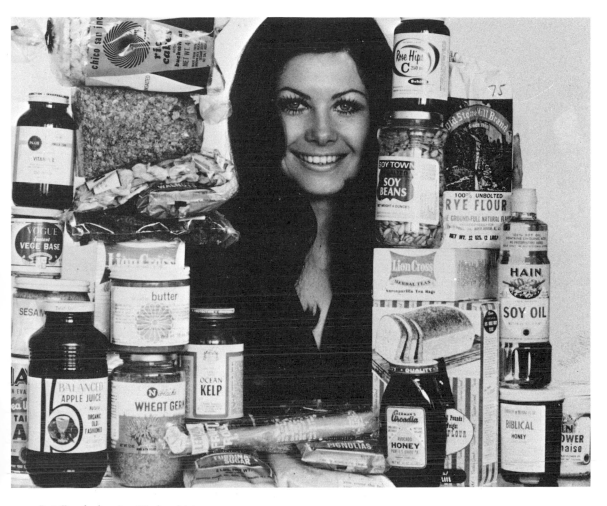

Pat Barrie is a health food-ist. Wheat germ is a part of her breakfast every morning, seven days a week.

CHAPTER · 14

The Wonderful
World
of Health Foods

Fifty-seventh Street in Manhattan is one of New York City's great crosstown thoroughfares, and one of my favorite streets in the whole world. On the east side are some of the city's smartest shops: florists that are veritable jungles of flowers, plants, and trees . . . fur salons where mink *really* is commonplace . . . banks that look more like diplomatic residences . . . beauty salons that look like pink-and-white pavilions. But cross Fifth Avenue and head west and you enter another world—very Middle European and totally charming in its own distinctive way. There's Carnegie Hall, the famous Russian Tea Room, the Art Students League, a clutch of bookstores—and one of my very favorite health food stores. Whenever I can, I drop in to browse around and, when I can squeeze in, I climb up on a stool and enjoy a counter lunch. A big glass of a freshly squeezed vegetable juice, a healthful salad with little squares of whole grain bread, and yogurt for dessert. I say *when I can,* because almost invariably there's standing room only, with not a few of my model friends already in line. For we all know the value of health foods, and so should you.

Model Diane Rystadt knows as much about health foods as I think it's possible for anyone to know without being a bona fide nutritionist. She snubs sugar in favor of honey for sweetening, bypasses soft drinks in place of fruit juices; insists on brown rice, which is rice in its natural state with much more protein then the bleached (and only 100 calories to a whole cup!). Of course, Diane has a juicer at home and she's a whiz at whipping up all sorts of health cocktails. Fresh carrot, apple, and orange. Spinach, lemon, and tomato. *Lipsmackers* and positively loaded with vitamins!

Lemon-blonde Gunilla Knutson, another Wilhelmina model, made the cover of *Life* magazine—that smashing issue devoted to the national popularity of health foods. Gunilla is famous as television's "Take it all off" girl.

108

And, of course, more and more men—the head-turning kind who exude animal vitality—are health food enthusiasts, too. When Danny Kaye is in New York, he's certain to drop by Brownie's, a sensational health food store and restaurant at Union Square. International hair stylist Vidal Sassoon who, over 40, weighs the same as he did at 25, is practically the Billy Graham of the health food cult. Every morning the dynamic Vidal follows his breakfast juice with a cup of yogurt to which he's added one raw egg, five tablespoons of wheat germ, and one tablespoon of honey. "That's where it's at," says Vidal, spooning the last dollop.

Now, suppose you come browsing with me through a health food store and we'll take an alphabetic tour of the shelves.

ASCORBIC ACID tablets are a source of vitamin C and considered a year-round insurance against colds. No wonder most models always have a supply handy. Red-tipped nose and watery eyes add up to canceled bookings. Some girls take a 250-milligram tablet with each meal. I prefer a 500-milligram tablet after breakfast and another just before retiring. Either way, I urge you to add a total of 1,000 milligrams of ascorbic acid to your diet *every* day.

BREWER'S YEAST is regarded as a wonder food, and it's easy to see why: it's been found to contain *17 vitamins,* including the entire B family. Yet brewer's yeast is almost zero as far as fat, sugar, and starch are concerned. The powdered form can be bought in a jar and added to fruit juices and tomato juice. If your complexion is anything less than radiant, I strongly recommend that you add this complete food to your diet.

CALCIUM TABLETS One day while taking something or other off one of the shelves in a health food store I had wandered into, I found myself *vis-à-vis* Tanya Leveau, who happened to be in one of the other aisles. And what was she buying? Calcium tablets. She takes them regularly, regarding them as essential to strong teeth, bones, and nails.

109

HERBS Cooking with herbs is a healthful way to put tang into your foods without having to resort to artificial flavorings. You can use them with both cooked foods and raw foods. Herbs also nourish internal organs and stimulate normal blood circulation. Buy your herbs in small quantities, since once their container has been opened and they're exposed to the air, they begin to lose strength.

There are so many herbs that I couldn't possibly list them all here (a good basic cookbook will, however), but here's a partial list with some suggestions on how to use them:

Lemon thyme in your tea in place of lemon.

Mint leaves chopped into your fruit salad. Ditto *peppermint leaves.*

Basil sprinkled on all tomato dishes (especially tasty with a tomato and lettuce salad), scrambled eggs, and Manhattan clam chowder.

Celery Salt does wonders sprinkled over chicken croquettes, on cauliflower, or in bouillon.

Oregano in a salad or as a poultry seasoning for stuffing.

HONEY is nature's sugar. It acts as a natural laxative. And since it enters the bloodstream directly, it earns the right to be labeled an *instant energy food.* Use it instead of sugar. Put a dollop of it on top of your grapefruit. On your toast instead of butter. On waffles. Add it to a glass of warm water and lemon juice and drink it down.

KELP is a sea vegetable, a form of seaweed that is a fantastic source of iodine. An insufficient supply of iodine spells overweight, tiredness, and even mental depression. You can buy kelp in tablet form and, like the rosy-cheeked youngsters of Norway, pop them down like candy. It's also available in powdered form to be used as a seasoning in soups.

SOYBEANS are rich in lecithin, a natural product found in the cells of most plant and animal life. Lecithin is an emulsifier of fat, and has been found to reduce the cholesterol level in the blood. It acts like a natural tranquilizer. Any wonder, then, that Orientals call the soybean their *holy* bean? You can buy soybean oil capsules in any health food store, but did you know you can grow your own soybeans? Here's how: Line a dish with moistened cotton. Put soybean seeds in it and put the dish in a sunny spot. Every day add a little water and in about four days your soybeans will start to sprout. When the sprouts are an inch high, eat them as a salad or sprinkle them over cooked vegetables.

SUNFLOWER SEEDS are literally packed with iron, calcium, iodine, and vitamins B, D, and E. Lovely thing is you can eat them for a between-meal snack. You can also toss them into salads, add them to yogurt, and sprinkle them into soups. And yes, you can toss them into a health drink you might be preparing in your electric blender. They're as versatile as they are nutritious.

WHEAT GERM is the heart of the kernel, the most nutritious part of the wheat. It's rich in protein, calcium, iron, and vitamins B and E. You can enjoy it as a cereal, mix it with pancake or waffle batter, add it to fruit juice, sprinkle it over fresh fruit, use it as a topping on salads, casseroles, and puddings. Gaylord Hauser reports that the dazzling Marlene Dietrich eats wheat germ—and yogurt—"until they come out of her ears."

I suggest that you invest in a giant jar and then try some of the recipes at the end of this chapter, which will give you an opportunity to put this remarkable food to work in your diet in any number of delicious ways.

YOGURT deserves a chapter all its own. Yogurt is so nutritious, my own refrigerator is never without it, and when I lunch at my health food store it's my favorite dessert. Yogurt consumption has increased by over 500 percent in the United States during the last decade. But more yogurt is eaten in food-conscious France than in any other country in the world!

I believe nutritionist Adelle Davis summed it all up when she wrote: "People who eat yogurt almost invariably become enthusiastic about it, often notice a marked pick-up in health following its use. This milk has long been the principal food of the Bulgarians and is considered responsible for their unusual health. These people are noted for retaining the characteristics of youth to a late age, and for unusually long lives. The 1930 census showed that there were over 1,600 Bulgarians over 100 years of age to every million of population compared to only nine persons in America. Moreover, it is said that baldness and white hair are almost unknown in Bulgaria."

Between sunflower seeds and wheat germ, I think I should have listed *Wanda.* Not a health food but a healthy, lovely ex-model who spreads health to droopy New Yorkers in summer via her "Super

111

Fruit Special" food cart. Wearing a frilly white apron and a wide-brimmed straw chapeau, "Wandering Wanda," as she calls herself, stocks her mobile cart with such healthful goodies as luscious fruits and berries served up with yogurt, honey, shortcake, and a variety of juices. Wanda parks her colorful cart beneath a tree outside Central Park at noon and the line immediately starts forming. In my opinion, Wanda is a bona fide pioneer in the health food movement.

I find the more I learn about these wonder foods, the more fascinated I become. It's the magic that comes from learning. On my bookshelves both in the city and in the country, I have the complete works of Gaylord Hauser and Adelle Davis. The pages are well thumbed, for I turn back to these books again and again. Not only are they full of facts about nutrition, but they're so interesting to read. So upbeat! So full of enthusiasm for living!

If you live nowhere near a health food store but would like to know more about the foods they offer, for just 25 cents you can order a catalog that will give you a complete rundown. Write to All Diet Foods, Inc., 16 West 40th Street, New York, N. Y. 10018. (Since these are inflationary times we live in, may I suggest you drop them a card first to make absolutely certain of the price before ordering?)

RECIPES USING WHEAT GERM

MAIN DISHES

Braised Beef Rolls

Fruit Stuffing
¼ cup butter or margarine
¼ cup chopped onion
½ cup chopped celery
½ cup peeled, chopped apple
¼ cup raisins
1½ cups soft bread crumbs
¾ cup Kretschmer Wheat Germ
¼ teaspoon salt
¼ cup water

Melt butter in a skillet. Add onion and celery. Sauté until onion is soft but not brown. Stir in the remaining dry ingredients. Add water, toss lightly with a fork, and set mixture aside.

Beef Rolls
  2 pounds flank steak
     Instant meat tenderizer
  2 tablespoons butter
  ½ teaspoon salt
  1 can (10½ ounces) consomme or beef
       broth
  1 cup water
  3 tablespoons unsifted flour

Tenderize the meat according to package directions. Spread it with
Fruit Stuffing (above) to within ½ inch of each edge. Press stuffing
firmly into place. Roll up the meat lengthwise. Cut it into desired
number of rolls. Skewer or tie each roll securely with heavy string.

Melt butter in a skillet. Brown beef rolls in butter, turning as necessary. Sprinkle with salt.

Combine consomme and water. Pour ½ cup of consomme mixture
over beef rolls. Cover and simmer until meat is tender (about 2
hours). Turn occasionally.

Remove the beef rolls from skillet onto a warm serving platter.
Blend remaining consomme mixture and flour. Stir into drippings
in the skillet to make gravy. Cook until thickened. Serve the gravy
over the beef rolls. (6-8 servings)

Ham Loaf
  3 cups (1½ pounds) ground ham
  1 cup (½ pound) ground pork
  ¾ cup Kretschmer Wheat Germ
  ½ cup finely chopped onion
  ¾ cup milk
  ½ cup catsup
  2 eggs
  1 teaspoon Worcestershire sauce

Combine all ingredients in a large bowl, mixing well. Press firmly into
9 X 5 X 3-inch loaf pan. Bake at 350° for 1 hour and 15 minutes.
Let it stand in the pan 10 minutes, then turn it out onto a serving
plate. Slice and serve with creamed vegetables, mustard, or tomato
sauce. (6-8 servings)

Wheat-Meat Loaf

```
2   cups (1 pound) ground beef
1   cup (½ pound) ground pork
1   cup Kretschmer Wheat Germ
¾   cup tomato juice, catsup, or milk
1   egg
1   tablespoon Worcestershire sauce
1   tablespoon chopped onion
1   teaspoon prepared mustard
½   teaspoon salt
```

Combine all ingredients in a large bowl, mixing well. Shape firmly into a round, flat loaf about 1 inch thick. Place it in a heavy 10-inch skillet or electric frypan. Cut almost through the meat loaf with a knife into desired number of pie-shaped servings.

Prepare Onion Gravy (below). Pour over the meat. Cover and simmer for 30 minutes or until meat is done as desired. (6-8 servings)

Onion Gravy
```
1   envelope dry onion soup mix
2   tablespoons unsifted flour
2   cups boiling water
```

Combine soup mix and flour. Stir to blend. Add water gradually, mixing well.

Salmon Loaf

```
1   can (pound) salmon
½   cup chopped celery
¼   cup chopped onion
⅓   cup butter or margarine
3   tablespoons flour
1   teaspoon salt
¼   teaspoon pepper
2   cups milk
4   eggs, slightly beaten
½   cup Kretschmer Wheat Germ
2   tablespoons chopped parsley
1   tablespoon lemon juice
```

114

Drain the salmon and save the liquid. Remove skin and bones. Sauté celery and onion in butter until onion is tender. Remove celery and onion from the pan and set aside.

Blend flour, salt, and pepper into the melted butter in the same pan until smooth. Add the milk all at once. Cook over medium heat until mixture thickens, stirring constantly.

Remove 1 cup of sauce for Hot Tartar Sauce (below). Place in saucepan. Combine remaining sauce with salmon, salmon liquid, celery, onion, and remaining ingredients. Mix well. Pour into greased, aluminum foil-lined, 9 X 5 X 3-inch loaf pan. Bake at 350° for 45 minutes or until firm. Let stand in pan 10 minutes, then turn it out onto a serving plate. Slice and serve with Hot Tartar Sauce (below). (6 servings)

Hot Tartar Sauce

1 cup sauce (above)
¼ cup salad dressing
¼ cup pickle relish
1 tablespoon lemon juice

Measure all ingredients into a saucepan. Mix well. Heat slowly over low heat, stirring frequently.

SALADS AND VEGETABLES

Pineapple Cheese Salad

1 package (3 ounces) cream cheese, softened
3 tablespoons Kretschmer Wheat Germ
1 tablespoon pineapple syrup
6 slices pineapple, drained
6 lettuce leaves
  Salad dressing, if desired

Combine cream cheese, wheat germ, and pineapple syrup. Mix well. Shape into 1-inch balls. Roll in additional wheat germ, if desired.

Arrange each pineapple slice on a lettuce leaf. Top with a cheese ball. Serve with salad dressing, if desired. (6 servings)

115

Vegetable Nut Loaf

1   cup diced carrots
1   cup diced celery
½   cup chopped onion
⅓   cup butter or margarine
¼   cup unsifted flour
1½ teaspoons salt
⅛   teaspoon pepper
1½ cups milk
1   cup grated American cheese
1   cup chopped pecans
¾   cup Kretschmer Wheat Germ
3   eggs, slightly beaten

Sauté carrots, celery, and onion in butter until onion is tender. Stir in flour, salt, and pepper. Add the milk all at once. Cook over medium heat until mixture thickens, stirring constantly. Add cheese. Stir until melted. Stir in nuts, wheat germ, and eggs.

Pour into a greased, aluminum foil-lined, 9 × 5 × 3-inch loaf pan. Bake at 350° for 50 minutes or until firm. Let stand in pan 10 minutes, then turn it out onto a serving plate. Slice, and serve with Quick Cheese Sauce (below). (6-8 servings)

Quick Cheese Sauce
1   can (10½ ounces) condensed cheese soup
½   cup milk

Combine the ingredients. Mix well. Heat slowly over low heat, stirring frequently.

DESSERTS

Lemon Tea Cookies

1   cup unsifted flour
¾   cup Kretschmer Wheat Germ
1½ teaspoons baking powder
½   teaspoon salt

¾ cup sugar
½ cup butter or margarine
1 egg
2 teaspoons grated lemon rind
2 tablespoons lemon juice
1 egg white, lightly beaten
   Granulated sugar

Measure flour, wheat germ, baking powder, and salt onto waxed paper. Stir well to blend. Cream sugar, butter, egg, lemon rind, and lemon juice thoroughly. Add blended dry ingredients to the creamed mixture. Mix well. Chill 1½-2 hours until firm.

Shape the dough into 1-inch balls. Dip tops in egg white, then in sugar. Place, sugar side up, on an ungreased baking sheet. Bake at 350° for 12-15 minutes. (4 dozen cookies)

Gingerbread

2 cups unsifted flour
½ cup Kretschmer Wheat Germ
½ cup sugar
1 teaspoon baking soda
¾ teaspoon salt
1½ teaspoons cinnamon
1½ teaspoons ginger
¼ teaspoon cloves
1 cup buttermilk
¾ cup light molasses
⅓ cup cooking oil or melted
      shortening
2 eggs

Measure dry ingredients into a bowl. Stir well to blend. Add liquid ingredients to the blended dry ingredients. Mix well. Pour into a well-greased 9-inch square pan. Bake at 350° for 35-40 minutes.

Cool on a rack 5 minutes before removing from pan. Serve warm with lemon sauce or whipped cream. (9 servings)

Streusel-Topped Apple Pie

Wheat Germ Pastry
¾ cup plus 2 tablespoons unsifted flour
2 tablespoons Kretschmer Wheat Germ
½ teaspoon salt
6 tablespoons shortening
2-3 tablespoons cold water

Measure flour, wheat germ, and salt into a bowl. Stir well to blend. Cut in half of the shortening until mixture resembles coarse meal, then remaining shortening until particles are the size of small peas. Add water a little at a time, mixing lightly with fork. Shape dough into a firm ball with your hands.

Roll out on a lightly floured cloth-covered board to 1/8-inch thickness. Place it loosely in 9-inch pie pan. Cut the dough 1 inch larger than the pan. Fold edge under. Moisten the rim of the pan. Flute edge.

Fill unbaked pastry with Apple Filling (below). Sprinkle evenly with Streusel Topping (below). Cover top of pie with aluminum foil. Bake at 425° for 30 minutes. Remove foil and bake 15-20 minutes more or until apples are tender. Serve warm or cool, as desired.

Apple Filling
¾ cup sugar
½ teaspoon cinnamon
¼ teaspoon nutmeg
5-6 large cooking apples, peeled and
          sliced thin

Combine sugar, cinnamon, and nutmeg. Mix this sugar mixture thoroughly with apples.

Streusel Topping
½ cup Kretschmer Wheat Germ
½ cup firmly packed brown sugar
¼ cup unsifted flour
½ teaspoon cinnamon
¼ cup butter or margarine

Measure dry ingredients into a bowl. Stir well to blend. Cut in butter with pastry blender until mixture resembles coarse meal.

BEVERAGES AND SNACKS

Hollywood Breakfast

¾ cup milk
½ cup orange juice
1 egg
1 teaspoon honey
2 tablespoons Kretschmer Wheat Germ

Blend all ingredients.

Pep Dip

2 cups (1 pint) commercial sour cream
½ cup Kretschmer Wheat Germ
¼ cup dried onion soup mix
   Milk (see note)
   Paprika, if desired

Measure sour cream, wheat germ, and soup mix into a bowl. Stir well to blend. Sprinkle with paprika before serving, if desired.

NOTE: If dip seems too thick, dilute with milk to desired consistency before serving.

Soup Snack

1 can (10½ ounces) condensed soup, any variety
1 can (10½ ounces) milk or water
¼ cup Kretschmer Wheat Germ

Combine soup and milk in a saucepan. Stir in wheat germ. Heat thoroughly. (3-4 servings)

Knowledgeable girls like model Randy Hague sip eight full glasses of clear water every day, crediting it with contributing to a flawless complexion *all over.*

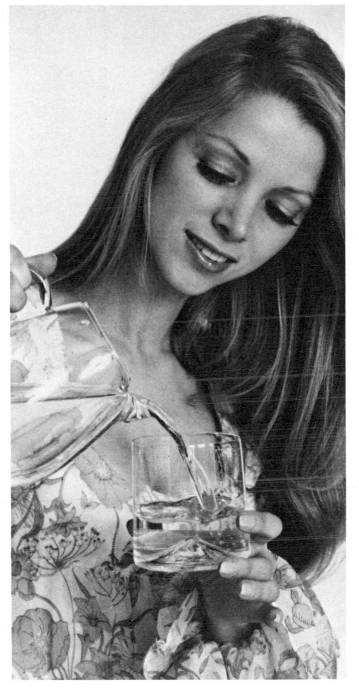

CHAPTER · 15

The Wonderful
World of Water

In the sixties, New York City had a severe water shortage. So severe, in fact, even the poshest restaurants stopped serving it with meals, except for a discreet splash or two for someone who had a pill to swallow. I was shattered. For I consider water to be a beauty essential—internally and externally. When the crisis was over I felt like celebrating and I did. Not with a glass of champagne, but with a pitcher of crystal clear water.

I drink a minimum of six glasses a day. It is, I think, the great cleanser, helping to eliminate body wastes. Poor elimination can result in a bumpy, muddy-looking complexion. Every time I see what a shower of rain does for the flowers and grass around our home in the country, I'm reminded that that is what drinking water does for one's complexion.

I love water so much I don't bathe in it, I cradle in it! It has such a soothing effect on the nerves that I regard a bath as much more than a beauty ritual. It's therapeutic as well. It relaxes you. It soothes you. It pampers you. And so it should be very much a part of your diet plan.

Every model appears to have her favorite bath. Mine is an every-night love affair with water.

Oleda's Hot Water, Iced Tea Beauty Treatment

1. First take your phone off the hook (unless you can resist the urge to pop out of a tub and answer it; I can't). If you're alone, make up your mind that the doorbell may ring, and if it does, well you'll just let it ring. The next half hour is going to be all yours. That lovely thought alone is almost enough to relax you.
2. Prepare a glass of iced tea. Then, with the glass in hand, walk slowly to your bathroom. Don't rush on

122

any account. For perhaps the first time all day, time is of no importance.

3. Place your glass of iced tea by the tub. Next to it, a bottle of baby oil. Start the hot water pouring into the tub. Let the water be as hot as you can possibly stand it. Add a few drops of bubble bath (or a few drops of liquid dishwater soap).

4. While your tub is filling, start removing your makeup following the *deep-down* cleansing method we've already discussed in Chapter 5.

5. Once your face and throat are feeling spic-and-span, step into your tub and relax. The hot water faucet should still be pouring—lightly, continuously—and that, pet, should be the only sign of action. Remain motionless up to your pretty shoulders in hot water and sparkling bubbles—at least 5 or 10 minutes. Wash with soap and cloth; put the used soapy cloth in the *sink*. Then dip into your tub again. After a few minutes, reach for your iced tea and sip ever so slowly. You'll soon start perspiring and your face will become pleasantly flushed. Sip and relax. Sip and relax. Let a good twenty minutes ooze by. (Much as I hate to mention it, you may want to have a clock nearby. More than twenty minutes in a hot tub could be weary-making and you want to be a rested beauty, *not* a weak one.) With the top of your bath water gurgling out via the top overflow drain of the tub, your water is still clean, and you're feeling light, airy and 100 percent carefree.

6. When those glorious, do-nothing twenty minutes have finally passed, reach for your bottle of baby oil. Tip in several drops. Turn the hot water off now, lie back and slowly massage some of that delicately oiled water into your skin.

7. Step out of your tub and towel dry.

8. Whenever possible, I lie down for the next five to ten minutes, with cold-water-soaked cotton pads pressed over each eyelid.

Vernice's Milk Bath

Shades of Cleopatra. And of Anna Held, the turn-of-the-century Follies beauty, an exquisite French doll of a woman with a complexion like a camellia, who was said to immerse herself in a tub of creamy milk every night of her life. Vernice Gabriel, very much a seventies girl with a Grade A complexion all over, adores her foamy milk baths, too.

There are, of course, milk bath powders available at the cosmetic counters at most drug and department stores, but Vernice, a redheaded beauty, has never bothered trying any of them. She simply stops by her friendly neighborhood grocer's and picks up a packet of powdered skim milk. With one of her long, protein-rich fingernails she slits it open and pours the contents into her tub which is already filling up with hot water. In practically no time at all, her bath water is being whipped into a creamy foam, very much like pure snow that's been suddenly and miraculously heated. Sheer luxury! Vernice follows her milk bath with a clear water rinse, and then towel dries. It's pure illusion, she admits, but immediately after her milk bath her skin looks *pearlized*.

Heather's Mint Pick-Up Bath

Heather Hazell is one of the most vital people I know. Simply sitting in the blue-and-white drawing room of her apartment in the United Nations Plaza (her neighbors include Truman Capote, the David Susskinds, and Johnny Carson), she exudes Rosalind Russell-type energy—the extraordinary kind that once prompted an admirer to note "Roz doesn't take vitamins. They take her!"

Heather has so much *joie de vivre,* you could sit in the ballroom of, say, the giant Americana hotel, at a table that's practically a city block away from the fashion runway, and Heather would still reach you. Even from that distance you would spot the energy in her walk, for example, which on the runway is more like a fashionable prance. Such dynamic vitality isn't an accident. It's the result of sensible diet and wise, *very* wise beauty care. And Heather's daily bath is an important part of her beauty plan.

Her mint pick-up bath is a four-time-a-week ritual. Into a tub that's filling up with medium warm water ("Too hot and I want to go to

124

sleep"), Heather pours Estée Lauder's "Azuree," a green liquid with a very minty fragrance. In the tub, Heather uses Estée Lauder's vitamin-enriched Creme Soap, a two-faced bar containing vitamins A and D on one side, a rich cream on the other. First, she uses the vitamin side, massaging the soap into her skin with a good stiff bath brush. Next the cream side, and again Heather uses her bath brush to wake up circulation all over her body—back, arms, and especially elbows, where skin can often become dry and flaky. Stepping out of her mint-green tub, and after toweling herself dry, Heather rubs herself all over with Estée Lauder's amber-colored body conditioner that boasts both vitamins and herbs. Heather claims she feels so refreshed, she practically *tingles*!

Early in life, children learn to love their baths. It's play time. And you should love your bath, too. It's beauty time—your little corner of the day when you take time to pamper yourself, to feel like the most desirable woman in the world. And this ego-pampering is especially important during a time of dieting when, as we've said so often, you must never ever feel deprived.

Showers are nice—for men.

Baths—fragrant, bubbly, luxurious—are *essential* for girls of all ages.

Oleda with her husband, Stephen Baker, her father, Marvin Freeman, and son, David.

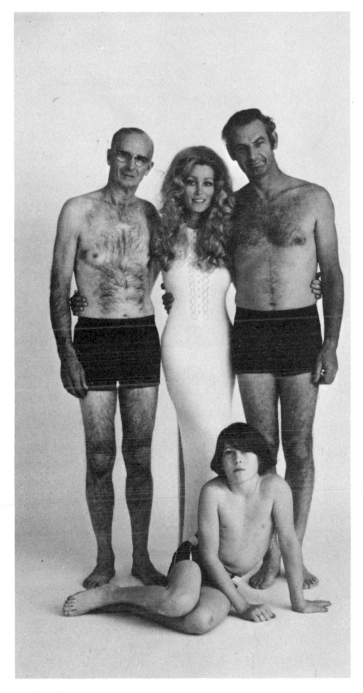

CHAPTER · 16

The Men
in Your Life

Or, as dear Mae West once so aptly put it, "The life in my men."
Brash, but true.

I have three charming men dressing up my life: my father, my
husband, and my son. All three are trim, athletic types. Not by
chance, but by plan. I must confess that I don't think I could
tolerate a fat man. If that makes me sound prejudiced, I plead guilty.
For I admire the opposite sex too much to want to see them eat
themselves into a state of obesity, one of the major contributing
factors in coronary disease.

The insurance actuaries figure it this way: The death rate of men
(of any age) who are 10 percent overweight averages 13 percent
higher overall than that of more slender men. The death rate of men
30 percent overweight is 42 percent greater than that of men of the
same age but of normal weight. Now, isn't that enough to make you
want to keep the men in your life slender?

My father, now in his sixties, is a handsome, rangy 6'2" and weighs
the same today as he did when I was a little girl. He did gain weight
around the "dangerous" age of 40, and how well I remember, first his
distress and then his gritty determination to do something about the
situation. And he *did*. He promptly cut down on starches, made it a
rule to swim almost every day (rather than once or twice a week),
and erected one chinning bar in the house and another out in the
garage. He lost his excess weight in a matter of weeks and never
gained it back. Well, over two decades have gone by and those two
chinning bars are still very much in evidence, and Dad rarely passes
them without hoisting himself up for a few chin-ups. He's still
swimming beautifully and, in fact, he long ago became a dedicated
scuba diver. Today there's not so much as an ounce of extra flesh on
his body. (But see for yourself. He's that distinguished-looking man
on the left in the "beefcake" picture of my three men.)

But Dr. Jean Mayer, professor of nutrition at Harvard University

128

and a champion of preventive medicine, maintains that the best solution to the overweight problem is to keep thin in the first place. And research scientists at Rockefeller University have suggested that due to overfeeding patterns in infancy and childhood some people simply have more fat cells than others. What a pity it is when a woman confuses excessive feeding with mother love!

Yet all too often a mother who is concerned about her daughter's figure is not at all concerned about her son's. She seems to think that somehow, magically, nature and sports will suddenly slim him down after years of too much cake, soda pop, and candy bars. How naïve! And if that doesn't happen—well, a boy isn't so sensitive about his appearance. Again, how naïve! And, unintentionally, how cruel!

"The overweight teen-ager is doomed to the role of wallflower at parties and to go through school dateless," says an eminent psychologist. "Even with members of their own sex, overweight teen-agers discover that their more attractive classmates do not want to be seen with them." Dr. Mayer regards obese youngsters as a persecuted minority.

Parents who want to save their children the humiliation of social exclusion because of excess weight simply can't begin too early to introduce them to proper eating habits which, if followed, will stay with them and help them grow to be happy, healthy, well-adjusted young adults. I certainly agree with the writer who declared, "Being fat is not only irresponsible, it's a distinct social liability." And perhaps saddest of all, the overweight teen-ager will develop such a negative self-image, will have so little ego, that, according to statistics, he will have an 80 percent chance of being fat after age 30.

I began my own program of "preventive medicine" with my son, David, when he was still an infant. My father had brought me up to believe that fresh air *plus* exercise *plus* proper diet *equals* bubbling good health, and I couldn't wait to get my baby started. Before he could even sit up, I was encouraging him to wrap his tiny fingers around my thumb and pull himself up. I wanted him to become aware of the strength he already had in those tiny arms! I started him on swimming lessons at the age of 4. By the time he was ready for school, he already enjoyed a glass of fresh fruit juice as much as a soda. When he grew to the gangly stage and seemed perennially

129

hungry, I introduced him to the fun of biting into a crunchy apple or juicy peach or a freshly scraped carrot as a between-meal snack. Today, at 14, David dives and swims the year round—in summer in the lake adjoining our country home, and in winter at the YMCA and the New York Athletic Club, which are a brisk walk from our New York apartment. David is an excellent skier, too, and the skipper of a 14-foot Sunfish sailboat, a fantastic little boat that keeps him on the alert every second. All in all, he's bursting with vitality but, I'm proud to say, not one excess pound. Very early in life, David developed that habit of liking what was good for him.

In fact, David has some of my missionary zeal when it comes to the subject of staying fit. And here, via tape recorder, are his own words on the subject:

"I never want to get fat because then I couldn't do a lot of things as well as I do now. Also, I wouldn't be able to wear the clothes I like, and I'd be teased by my friends. I feel sorry for fat kids. I wish they'd lose weight and see how much fun it is to be slim."

And certainly it's no secret that in today's youth-oriented society, a slender, taut figure is synonymous with youthfulness. An overweight man of 30 can look 40. But a slender man of 40 can look 30. And the difference may eventually show up in the size of their respective paychecks. The fact that some blue chip corporations have introduced fitness programs for their executives isn't simply a case of corporate philanthropy. It's a practical matter of dollars and sense. Many corporations are so sold on the theory that a slim, vital employee is more productive than a physically flabby one, that they are actually sponsoring executive programs on company time.

According to Dr. Jerry Saffer, staff psychologist at Chicago's Michael Reese Hospital Institute for Psychosomatic and Psychiatric Research and Training, the fat man often displays a tendency toward impulsiveness, which is not a desirable trait in the business executive. "There are economic gains for men when they lose excess weight," says another psychologist, who believes that as the pounds melt away, a man gains self-esteem. "Men often earn more money when they lose weight. The boss is so pleased with the weight loss that the man gets the promotion he should have had years ago."

Dr. Saffer believes, however, that the single most important factor

130

in a man's ability to lose weight and to keep it off is not career ambition, but "his wife's encouragement and interest." In short, never underestimate the power of a woman.

My husband is 6'4", and until the spring of 1970 he maintained his weight at a hard-muscled 185 pounds. Then, suddenly, the faint signs of a paunch. In his case it was in part the result of sitting too much, often in deep-cushioned office chairs that look so sensational in a plush advertising agency office but are enemies of good sitting posture. After being teased so long about my *twice*-daily weigh-ins, I began to find Steve standing behind me waiting for his turn on the family scale. Well, it was perfectly obvious that skiing (he's been on the slopes since age 5), swimming (he used to be one of the best in his native Hungary), and golf (he shoots in the middle 80s) simply weren't enough to melt away that incipient paunch. We were going to have to attack it *directly*. So I whipped up a mini-sized exercise regime following the justly famous "Royal Canadian Air Force Exercise Plan," and for the next several weeks Steve did fifteen minutes of exercise every morning before he shaved. We also *deemphasized* potatoes and bread and butter in his daily diet, and *emphasized* leafy green vegetables—that way snipping away at his daily caloric intake. Meantime, I'd popped into his newly decorated office and taken a look at the very elegant but very poorly designed chair he was spending so much of his time in. I decided it had to go—with his permission, of course. We replaced it with a straighter, harder chair. And on weekends in the country, Steve took to early-morning jogging before his golf game. *Result*: In less than four months, his weight was back to 185 and his stomach was washboard flat again. And I must admit I felt like a very helpful helpmate.

"It's interesting," observes Dr. Saffer, "that so many obese men have wives who are also fat." The wife who keeps ice cream and beer in the refrigerator, "for whatever reason, may unconsciously be sabotaging her husband's diet." And, I might add, her own happiness, too. For overweight is all too often a sign of a man's lack of interest in life—a cop-out. Dr. Howard Kurland, chief of psychiatry for the Veterans' Administration Research Hospital in Chicago, speculates that "the hyper-obese condition affords many protections . . . and restrictions of physical, social, and sexual activities."

131

So if your husband is slender, encourage him to stay that way. If he isn't, remember that a wife's encouragement and interest are essential to man's ability to lose weight. To be more specific . . .

1. Suggest he see his doctor, just as you did before starting on your diet. Notice, please, that I use the word *suggest*. Don't nag. Don't sound dictatorial. Express your interest in his well-being in the warmest, most womanly way you know.

2. When he has started his diet, use all your culinary know-how, all your imagination to make each meal you prepare a treat, not only to the taste buds but to the eye as well. Never allow a meal to look sparse. Never permit it to be rushed. Here are some rules to follow:

   Place on the table all the silverware needed for a full meal, even if all he'll need is a fork. A full service suggests there's no limit to what is being served.

   Before you and he sit down put everything else on the table that you'll need. Don't interrupt the pleasant, relaxed atmosphere by having to get up.

   A cloth napkin somehow gives a dieter a secure feeling. Add it to your table setting.

   Dress up your dishes! Put sliced hard boiled eggs around a meat platter, for instance. Sprinkle parsley into your soups. The more colorful they are, the more *appetizing* they look!

   Fill the table. Put carrot sticks in one container, celery stalks in another, and relishes, jams, and pickles in their separate containers, too. Add a platter of cold grapes. Even if you have only two slices of bread on the table, put them in a bread basket. Put crackers on small, colorful plates.

   Give him a choice of dressings for his salad. Have them all there on the table. He'll have so many decisions to make, so many dishes to reach for, he'll never have time to feel that he's being deprived!

3. Keep up his morale in the same way you've learned to keep up your own. For example, surprise him with a

132

pair of slacks in the waist size his diet is preparing him for—or a pair of colorful swim trunks he'll be proud to wear once he has his athletic physique back in working order. In other words, play to the Body Image he has in his mind's eye.

4. If he should fall off the diet wagon at any time, don't criticize—*sympathize*. But not too much. Just make it perfectly clear that you (of all people) understand, but that you (of all people) know that he won't slip again. How could he when he already looks so much more attractive?

5. Demonstrate your interest in the very best way I know—by your own example. Be a walking, talking advertisement for how much more fun life really is when you're slender!

Victoria Diaz knows how to enjoy dining out—no matter how plain or fancy—and still maintain her good health and trim figure.

CHAPTER · 17

How to Dine Out
Anywhere
and Still Lose
Weight

My husband is an advertising man, and entertaining is a necessary and very enjoyable part of his business. Often we have a dinner party in our apartment, but more often we take our guests to one of the glamorous restaurants that make dining out in New York such a pleasure.

Most of the chic restaurants have very cleverly engineered the entrance to their dining rooms so that there's space for only one guest at a time. You can make quite an effective entrance that way! The most stunning entrance I ever saw was Marlene Dietrich's at the Colony one winter's evening. In clinging black trimmed with sable, a tiny feathered hat over her silky blonde hair, la Dietrich paused for just a golden moment in the entrance . . . long enough to catch every eye . . . and then swept to her table. Breathtaking!

Now let me give you a sample or two of what I often order when dining out, determined as I am to eat well and stay slim enough to waft through the narrowest entrance.

Seafood is high in protein and slimming. And New York literally abounds in superb seafood restaurants. Here is one of my all-time favorite menus:

Shrimp cocktail with regular cocktail sauce
Clam broth
Steamed lobster with lemon and salt seasoning
Tossed green salad liberally sprinkled with carrots, and
    again with a lemon and salt seasoning
Cantaloupe
Tea

A feast! And yet that delicious dinner contains not a single fattening food. Did I deny myself? Not at all. I did without butter sauce with my lobster, but I didn't miss it and neither will you. Lemon and salt seasoning is so tasty! I chose steamed lobster but you may prefer your lobster broiled. In place of lobster, you can subsitute any fish you prefer.

Italian food is a particular weakness of mine. I've always enjoyed it, but never so much since I spent an entire summer modeling for Roman and Florentine couturiers—and dining under the stars at the very Italian hour of 10 P.M. in some of the most charming restaurants I've ever known. Fortunately, knowing something about food values, I didn't have to join the army of American models who, after a day of modeling, were absolutely famished but were so afraid of gaining weight that they sat at their table, surrounded by trays of mouth-watering foods, and picked away at a lettuce leaf. I ate and ate and ate.

Here is a sample of a typical dinner I enjoyed in Italy and still enjoy in many of New York's great Italian restaurants:

> Pickled mushrooms
> Consomme
> Veal Paillard (a flat rolled veal without bones)
> Tomato and oregano salad with oil and vinegar dressing
> Fruit bowl
> Espresso

No pasta? No parmigiana? That's right, no pasta, no parmigiana. A small price to pay when dining Italian-style.

Before flying home, I stayed a week in Paris. This was my vacation and I denied myself nothing. Absolutely nothing. I bought at St. Laurent and Givenchy. I scooped up hordes of treasure at Dior's boutique—glamorous small gifts for my sisters and friends. I had a facial, manicure, and pedicure at Elizabeth Arden's. And dinner (or late supper) every night at one of the four-star Parisian restaurants. My policy of deny-Oleda-nothing didn't stop there, either, as this menu proves:

137

Caviar
Onion soup
Broiled sweetbreads
Endive and braised celery
Demitasse

Still another evening, after a performance at the Paris Opera, my supper included a marvelous cucumber soup, a whole breast of chicken, and the most delicious asparagus I've ever tasted (and of course, with every meal I had some dry white wine).

So you see, you need have no fear that while dieting you must be a recluse. In fact, I think it's more important than ever that you get out and see friends and enjoy yourself. Under no circumstances should you feel like a martyr while slimming down.

When dining out, simply remember this rule: Explain to your waiter that whatever dish you order is to be prepared *without dressing or butter,* and there is to be *no fat or sauce.* (And yes, take care to skip the rolls and breads.)

And from that point on—enjoy, enjoy!

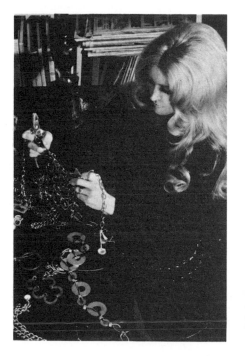

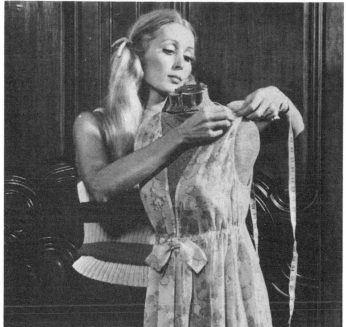

Some of the ways I deal boredom a body blow are

... by designing men's and women's jewelry that's fashioned of such trivia as bits of honest-to-goodness hardware;

... by sewing—a wise and wonderful hobby that I recommend for any woman who wants truly creative fashions that say something definitive about her;

... by painting pictures that art galleries show and art lovers buy. But you don't have to sell your work to get terrific enjoyment from doing it!

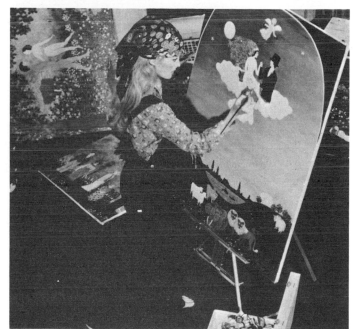

CHAPTER · 18

The Boredom Syndrome:
How to Beat It

I can't recall who the famous personality was who said, "I've never been bored," but I simply don't believe him. I would believe him, however, if he'd said, "I try never to permit myself to be bored." That's the difference, for we've all known boredom. Can't you remember, for instance, the boredom of a rainy day spent indoors when you were a child? It's the enterprising ones among us who, with maturity, decide never to permit themselves the anesthetic effect of boredom again. For it is like anesthesia. It saps one's physical energies, dulls the intellect, and dims awareness. Who can afford that?

I think of the remark Rose Kennedy made to a reporter who marveled at her resilience in the face of so much personal tragedy. She explained that she had simply made up her mind not to give in to sorrow, and so she involved herself with people and cultivated new interests. At 80, this remarkable woman talked of her plan to learn speed reading!

I speak of boredom now because you are practically certain to be threatened with it during your diet. Starting your diet at such a peak of enthusiasm, it's almost inevitable that at some point you experience a letdown. The thrill of stepping on the scale and discovering that you've dropped another pound will have lost a little of its excitement (imagine that!) and it may be one of those soggy Tuesdays when almost everything seems to lack luster. Prepare for this mid-diet droop and you'll beat it!

To do so, here's Oleda's Boredom Survival Kit:

FRESHEN UP YOUR OUTLOOK. How? By doing the unexpected. Say it's a wintry day with icicles coating the branches of your favorite tree. Start your spring housecleaning. After all, *who* ever said it has to be April to shake up the attic and clear out your hall closet?

You've been toying with the idea of investing in a smashing wig? *Now* is the time to buy it. A wig does for morale today what a new hat used to do day-before-yesterday.

140

Try a new restaurant. A new recipe. A new cologne or perfume. A new fashion color you've been too timid to try before.

Look up an old friend you've lost contact with.

In other words, shake up your corner of the world—and boredom will slip away.

START A NEW HOBBY. Pursue some subject that's always interested you but that you've just never had the time to cozy up to, or something that until now you felt you could never master. I recall a model I once worked with who one day startled us all in a photographer's studio when she picked up a pair of pliers and went to work—and expertly—on a piece of faulty hardware we were using as a prop. When we were back in the dressing room and slithering out of our dresses, I asked this exquisite creature, who had petite hands and l-o-n-g fingernails, how she had ever learned to be a Miss Fixit.

"I was terribly bored one day and decided to do something novel to snap me out of it," she explained. "I thought, 'What is costing me money that I could do myself?' I realized that getting things fixed around my apartment was costing me money in tips every time I called in the handyman. So I took myself off to the library next day, came home with a couple of good do-it-yourself books, and learned how to do things like fix a fuse, a leaky faucet—you know, all those little things that keep popping off."

Indeed I do know! I'm a Miss Fixit myself and have been for years: I simply don't have the patience to sit and wait for someone else to come around and do things for me. I've made minor repairs on our radio—even our portable television set. And I'm proud as a peacock of the 7-foot bookshelves I built for my son. After waiting weeks for a carpenter to show up, I measured the space in David's room set aside for the shelves, ordered the lumber, and went to work hammering and painting! I happen to be naturally adept with my hands, but if I weren't I can assure you that I'd learn to be. And so can *you*. It's creative, practical, and so much fun!

But if playing the glamorous "handyman" just doesn't appeal to you, there are countless other roads that will detour you from boredom by taking you outside yourself. And that's important, for let's face it, dieting can sometimes become more than a little narcissistic.

141

BONE UP ON INTERIOR DECORATION. Perhaps there's a nearby school with a course you can take, but if there isn't, there are scads of fascinating books available on the subject. How exciting and profitable it is, for example, to learn the ABCs of antique buying. And once you've mastered them, what fun it is to travel to out-of-the-way antique barns where really incredible finds are just waiting for the woman who knows how to recognize them.

I took a course in interior decoration at New York University. And Heather Hazell not only studied the subject but became so intrigued with it that she went on to get a license as a full-fledged interior decorator! Now when she isn't parading down a fashion runway, Heather is running around town buying beautiful furnishings for her clients.

A new-looking room can give you a new outlook on life. And it's so easy to learn how to freshen up a room for very little money—a slipcover in a cheery color, a clutch of sofa pillows in exciting patterns, a few green plants in snow-white pots ringing a table lamp. No wonder so many women consider a course in interior decoration or a few home-study books on the subject to be a fabulous investment!

LEARN THE ART OF MAKING YOUR OWN CLOTHES. I design and make many of my clothes for the very good reason that all too often I can't find what I want in the stores. I have a mannequin figure to fit my fabrics on, a good sewing machine, and a head full of designs I can't wait to turn into reality. I've even made shirts for my husband! And I would certainly encourage any girl about to enter the modeling profession to learn how to make her own clothes. That first year when you're getting started can be a lean one, yet you must always look chic. The smart girl who knows her way around a sewing machine can invest her money in superb fabrics and make her own clothes, copying fashions snipped directly from the pages of *Vogue* and *Harper's Bazaar*.

Remember, too, that you're soon going to want lots of new clothes to flatter your new figure. What better time than now to learn how to fill your closet in this highly creative and economical way! And once you've learned to sew, you can also alter all your much-too-large clothes down to your now smaller size.

142

MASTER A SECOND LANGUAGE. Enroll in a study course and let yourself go. I say let yourself go because it's very possible that when you last curled your tongue around a foreign verb, teaching methods were not as steamlined as they are today. Now learning a new language is, as it should be, a matter of ear appeal, rather than memorization and stuffy grammar.

You might also consider acquiring the long-playing records that teach a new language via the "hear and repeat" technique that was developed for the Army's "crash" language-training program. They're very effective. Or if you happen to know someone truly proficient in, say, French, and you're a snappy cook or seamstress or whatever, work up a fair exchange: one private French lesson for one private lesson in your specialty.

Any way you manage it, learning a new language is a thrill!

IMPROVE YOUR VOICE. A few years ago I met one of the most famous cover girls of all time, one of the truly topflight models back when Dior's New Look was The Look. She's still beautiful and slender, her blonde hair coiled in a French knot, her complexion flawless as porcelain breathtaking! Until she begins to talk. Then, what a disappointment—a flat, nasal voice bereft of charm.

Well, today, with television commercials a pot of gold for models, we simply must have voices that match our looks. And so should *every* woman. A less than charming voice is as much a charm killer as a pair of chapped hands or a chipped front tooth. All inexcusable.

Of course, there are classes to which one can go for speech training. The class that former stage star and singer Dorothy Sarnoff conducts in New York has as many men attending as women, and why not? A pleasant speaking voice is a business as well as a social asset. Many YWCAs also offer courses designed to show you how to cultivate a more charming speaking voice. And there are books on the subject in any public library. Or you can be your own tutor if you'll but learn to listen, objectively, to the sound of your own voice. Better yet, invest in a tape recorder. Turn it on and read aloud from a book, magazine, or newspaper; then play the tape back. It will be a revelation, I can promise you! Yes, and have a tape spinning when you're having just an everyday conversation with a friend or while

143

you're chatting on the telephone. In short, eavesdrop on YOU talking. Listen and be very critical. Do you really speak distinctly, articulating every word? Or do you race along, slurring syllables and dropping "G's" so that *going* is *goin'* and *coming* is *comin'*? And what about the quality of your voice? Is it pleasant to hear? Or is it thin and reedy? You can, you know, learn to pitch your voice lower. Then there's the matter of vocabulary. Even a charming voice loses something when speech is continually peppered with such clichés as "You know" and "I mean."

A lovely speaking voice can make even a plain woman seem beautiful. An unattractive voice, on the other hand, can—as I've already pointed out—rob even a great beauty of much of her allure. Only a few women are born with fabulous speaking voices; but with a little effort, any woman can acquire one.

BECOME A FLOWER CHILD. Not one of the barefoot-with-beads variety, but a poring-through-the-books, digging-in-the-earth garden variety. Plant the seeds for the most eye-appealing garden in town or, at the very least, the most imaginative floral centerpieces.

If you live in an apartment, learn all you can about plants, and fill your windowsills or decorate your rooms with some of the most offbeat greenery your friends have ever seen. I have what I like to think is the tallest rubber plant in New York—a stunning 18 feet high and still growing!

One of my model friends has become something of an expert on, of all things, *orchids*. There are books galore about flowers and plants, and my friend, a rather orchidaceous type herself, highly recommends her favorite, *Orchids and Serendipity* (Prentice-Hall, Inc.), in which author Hugo Freed writes: ". . . to me, one of the nicest things about entering the world of orchids is the people you meet. My friends and associates include truck drivers, dentists, carpenters, airline pilots, housewives, retired military officers, lawyers, doctors, representatives from almost every other type of trade or profession you can call to mind."

TRY PETIT POINT. I know girls whose hair is done by Mr. Kenneth himself, who trip to Europe twice a year for the fashion collections, and who regard mink as a commonplace fur. What do they have in

144

common with the girl who lives on a budget and takes her lunch at a drugstore counter? *Petit point.* It's challenging, fascinating, relaxing, and, I think, well worth your investigating. There are excellent books available on this subject too. Many models enjoy petit point and have walls full of pictures and sofas full of pillows they've designed.

TAKE AN ART COURSE. Painting is my love, and I'm serious about it. When the last page of this manuscript is finished, I'll go back to finishing enough canvases for my first one-woman exhibition. By now, I imagine, just about everyone knows how many men and women in all walks of life have found painting or sketching or sculpting to be a wonderful emotional outlet.

DO VOLUNTEER WORK. There's so much you can do and so many people who need you. In a city, of course, the number of opportunities is enormous, and although in a small town the opportunities may be fewer, the rewards are no less rich. Working unselfishly for someone else is, in my opinion, one of the greatest cosmetic aids any woman can enjoy. It's every bit as flattering as that *in-love* look that drenches even the plainest woman in beauty.

Whichever road you choose to take you away from boredom, it will be an exciting one. The new, the challenging, is always an adventure. And now that you're about to step out with a svelte new figure, why not have a matching personality? A new hobby, a new interest, is the best exercise I know for a personality that may have developed its own kind of middle-age spread.

Who says a dieter has to nibble on dry crackers at dessert
time? Not model Pamela
Berkin, who proves that you
don't, via this dessert dazzler
that adds up to deliciously
few calories.

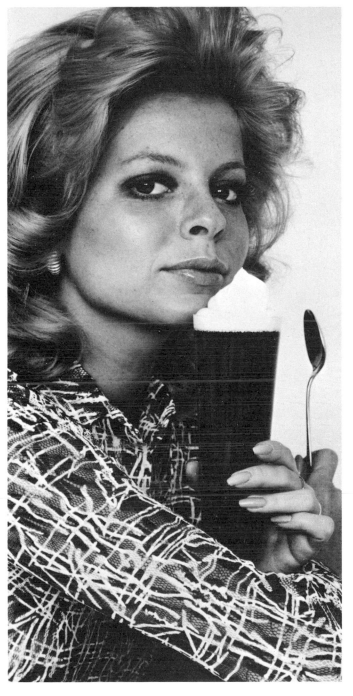

CHAPTER · 19

Delicious Things to Do With Food While Dieting

Just because a dish is short on calories, there's no reason why it must be short on eye appeal, too—not when there are scads of ways you can add dashes of color that give even the "skinniest" recipe a voluptuous personality. A curl of red pepper. A pimiento. A sprig of watercress. Alluring toppings like that can dress up any dish. And then, of course, there are those dishes that by themselves are eye-catchers *par excellence*. Here is a collection of my all-time favorites:

Sliced Beef en Gelée

      6 slices cold roast beef or pot roast
     ½ teaspoon thyme
     ½ teaspoon basil
     ½ teaspoon salt
         Dash of freshly ground black pepper
      1 carrot, sliced
     ½ green pepper in strips
      2 envelopes unflavored gelatine
   1½ cups cold water
      2 cans condensed consomme
      1 teaspoon Worcestershire sauce
         Dash of cayenne pepper

Overlap slices of beef in a shallow serving dish. Sprinkle with thyme, basil, salt, and black pepper. Garnish with carrot slices and green pepper strips. Soften gelatine in ½ cup of cold water. Bring 1 can consomme to a boil and add it to the gelatine, stirring until the gelatine is dissolved. Add the remaining can of cold consomme, 1 cup of cold water, Worcestershire sauce, and a few grains of cayenne pepper. Cool until the gelatine mixture is syrupy (approximately 25 minutes). Pour the mixture over the beef slices and chill in the refrigerator for at least 2 hours or until the gelatine is set. (6 servings)

Tongue in White Wine Aspic

1⅓ pounds sliced cooked tongue
    Stuffed olives
2 envelopes unflavored gelatine
½ cup cold water
2 cans condensed consomme
1⅓ cup dry white wine

Overlap slices of tongue in two rows along each side of a shallow serving dish. Arrange a row of stuffed olives in the center. Soften gelatine in ½ cup of cold water. Bring 1 can of consomme to a boil and add it to the gelatine, stirring until the gelatine is dissolved. Stir in the wine and remaining can of cold consomme. Cool for 25 minutes, until the wine and gelatine mixture is slightly syrupy. Pour over the tongue and chill in the refrigerator for at least 2 hours or until the wine aspic has set. (6 servings)

Low-Calorie Dressing

1 cup salad oil
1½ cups garlic vinegar
3½ tablespoons grated lemon rind
3½ tablespoons chopped parsley
    Freshly ground black pepper
1 tablespoon minced fennel
1 tablespoon celery salt
1 teaspoon oregano
1 teaspoon ground chervil
1 teaspoon dry mustard

Combine all ingredients in a jar or cruet. Cover. Shake well before using. Makes 3 cups.

Vegetable Salad Bowl

    2 medium tomatoes, sliced
    ½ cup cooked snap beans
    ½ cup cooked kidney beans
    ½ cucumber, sliced
    1 zucchini squash, sliced
    ⅓ cup sliced raw mushrooms
       Broccoli flowerets
    2 carrots, in thin strips
    1 cup radish slices
    1 onion, sliced
       Mixed greens
       Salad dressing

Marinate tomatoes and cooked vegetables in the refrigerator for at least 4 hours in French or low-calorie dressing. Drain and save marinade. Arrange marinated and raw vegetables on a bed of mixed greens. When ready to serve, use marinade as dressing. (6 servings)

Veal and Chicken Salad

    1 cup cooked veal strips
    1 cup cooked chicken strips
    ⅓ cup sliced celery
    2 medium apples, cubed
    6 stuffed olives, sliced
    1 tablespoon minced chives
       Pistachio nuts
       Mixed greens
       Salad dressing

Arrange veal, chicken, celery, apples, and olives on a bed of mixed greens. Decorate with chives and a few pistachio nuts. When ready to serve, toss with French or sweet and sour dressing. (6 servings)

150

Bouillabaisse Salad

1	cup cooked crabmeat
¾	cup cooked lobster meat
½	pound cooked shrimp
1	cup cooked whitefish
2	tomatoes, sliced
8	ripe olives, halved
	Mixed greens
	Salad dressing

Arrange crab, lobster, shrimp, whitefish, and tomatoes on a bed of mixed greens. Garnish with olives. To serve, toss with classic French or hot spice dressing. (6 servings)

Sweet and Sour Meatballs

5	thin bread slices, cut into ½-inch cubes
½	cup milk
1	egg
2	pounds ground round steak
1¼	teaspoons salt
⅛	teaspoon pepper
⅛	teaspoon monosodium glutamate
⅛	teaspoon garlic salt
¼	cup flour
2	tablespoons salad oil
¾	cup cold water
1	8-ounce can tomato sauce
¼	cup white vinegar
⅓	cup granulated sugar
½	cup sweet gherkin chunks
1	can (13½ ounces) pineapple chunks, drained
2	small green peppers, cut in bite-size pieces
1	carrot, sliced diagonally

In a large bowl, combine bread cubes, milk, and egg. Let stand for 5 minutes. Then, with a fork, press together until bread is wetted through; add ground steak, pepper, monosodium glutamate, and

151

garlic salt. With your hand, knead this meat mixture until well mixed; then shape into approximately 40 meatballs and, one by one, roll them in the flour; shake off excess flour and set aside.

In hot salad oil, in large skillet over medium heat, brown meatballs until light golden. Then remove to paper toweling. Wipe remaining salad oil from skillet, then put meatballs back in skillet with water, tomato sauce, vinegar, sugar, 1 teaspoon salt, and sweet gherkins. Set aside 10 pineapple chunks and add the rest to meatballs. Simmer uncovered over low heat, turning often, for 12 minutes or until about $\frac{2}{3}$ of the liquid in the meatball mixture evaporates.

Meanwhile, in 1 tablespoon salad oil in medium saucepan over medium heat, sauté green peppers, carrot slices, and ¼ teaspoon salt until tender-crisp (about 3 to 5 minutes). Then, add half of green pepper and carrot mixture to meatballs, and stir until heated through. Spoon into a large serving bowl, then top with reserved pineapple chunks and the rest of green pepper and carrot mixture. (8 servings)

Sirloin-Shrimp Dinner Platter

10 boned sirloin steaks, each
        2¼ × 2¼ × 1½ (about 3 pounds)
1 teaspoon instant meat tenderizer
   White pepper
   Ginger
   Salad oil
1 teaspoon salt
10 bacon strips
   Toothpicks
3 10-ounce packages frozen
     whole-kernel corn
   Dash garlic salt
30 large shelled, deveined shrimp
2 medium onions, sliced
3 10-ounce packages frozen green
     peas and pearl onions
1 clove garlic, minced
   Parsley for garnish

152

In a bowl, sprinkle steaks with meat tenderizer, dash of white pepper, dash of ginger, 1 teaspoon salad oil and dash of garlic salt. Toss and refrigerate 2 hours.

In medium bowl, sprinkle shrimp with salt, dash of white pepper, and dash of ginger. Toss well. Preheat broiler. Wrap a bacon strip around the sides of each steak and secure with toothpicks. Broil the steaks, 4 inches from heat, about 7 minutes on each side.

Start cooking the corn and the peas. Meanwhile, in 3 tablespoons salad oil in hot skillet, sauté onions and garlic till soft. With a slotted spoon, remove onions and discard garlic. In the same oil, sauté shrimp until pink and tender. Return onions, stirring until heated. To serve: on heated large platter arrange shrimp, peas and onions, corn, and steaks (remove picks) in rows. Garnish with parsley sprigs. (10 servings)

Apple Dessert Pancakes

     2 eggs
     ⅔ cup milk
     1 tablespoon melted shortening
     ¼ teaspoon salt
        Granulated sugar
     ⅔ cup sifted all-purpose flour
     3 small apples
        Butter or margarine

In a blender or electric mixer, beat eggs thoroughly. Add milk, shortening, salt, and 1 teaspoon sugar. Then beat once more. Add flour and beat until you have a smooth batter. Pare and core apples. Slice very thinly into at least 16 slices.

Heat 1 teaspoon butter in a 7-inch skillet. Place 2 apple slices in it and sauté until tender-crisp. Then, with ¼ cup measuring cup as a scoop, pour scant ¼ cup batter over apple slices. Tilt skillet to spread batter over the bottom of it. Cook pancake until brown on bottom. With narrow spatula, loosen sides and under part of apple slices. Now invert pancake into another hot buttered small or large skillet and sauté until underside is golden brown. Then slip onto a square of waxed paper on

153

a wire rack. In the same way continue making pancakes, placing each on the waxed paper square, then piling one on top of another.

Now remove each pancake from waxed paper, carefully fold it in half, then lay, in overlapping row, down center of a cookie sheet or stainless steel platter. Set aside.

Sprinkle pancakes with 2 tablespoons sugar; broil until hot and bubbly. If broiled on cookie sheet, transfer to heated platter for serving. (8 servings)

Lamb and Carrot Meatballs

1	pound lean lamb shoulder, ground
1	cup finely grated carrots
1	small onion, finely chopped
¼	cup dried bread crumbs
1	egg
1½	cups water
2	teaspoons salt
¼	teaspoon black pepper
½	teaspoon basil
¼	teaspoon thyme
2	tablespoons butter or margarine
2	tablespoons flour

In a large bowl, mix lamb, carrots, onion, bread crumbs, egg, salt, pepper, basil, and thyme; form into 8 balls. In butter or margarine, in a large skillet sauté lamb balls until well browned.

Meanwhile, in small bowl, slowly add water to flour, stirring well. Stir flour-water mixture into the skillet with the gravy until it is smooth, then cover and simmer 45 minutes. Arrange meatballs on a small platter. Skim fat from gravy, then pour gravy over meatballs sparingly and serve the rest in a pitcher. (4 servings)

154

Potted Shoulder of Veal

1	4-pound boned shoulder of veal
2	teaspoons seasoned salt
¼	teaspoon seasoned pepper
½	teaspoon thyme
3	tablespoons salad oil
1⅓	cups canned chicken broth
4	large pared potatoes, quartered
1½	pounds fresh green beans, cleaned and left whole
	Chopped parsley for garnish

At least 2 hours before serving, unroll shoulder of veal, trim away extra fat from meat, and sprinkle meat with seasoned salt, seasoned pepper, and thyme. Roll it up again and tie with string.

In hot salad oil, in large Dutch oven, brown veal on all sides. Add chicken broth and simmer, covered, about 1½ hours.

Now add quartered potatoes and cook for 10 minutes, then add green beans and continue cooking until both vegetables and veal are tender. Thinly slice the veal into serving portions. To serve: arrange veal on platter with potatoes and green beans around it. Spoon some of the gravy over all, serving the rest in a gravy boat. Sprinkle with parsley. (8 servings)

Scallopini à la Marsala

1	pound veal round, cut about ¼ inch thick for scallopini
¼	cup flour
1	teaspoon seasoned salt
	Dash of black pepper
1⅔	tablespoons butter or margarine
¼	cup dry Marsala wine
¼	cup water

155

If necessary, cut meat into pieces about 3 inches square. Cut away any fell (the white skin or connective tissue) or fat from meat. With a mallet or heavy wooden bowl, pound veal into very thin slices—about 1/8 inch thick.

On a sheet of waxed paper, mix flour, seasoned salt, and pepper. Dip both sides of veal into the mixture and shake off excess.

In butter or margarine, in a large skillet, quickly sauté veal until lightly browned, removing pieces from the pan as they are done (about one minute on each side). When all meat is cooked, return it to the skillet; add Marsala and water. Cook, gently scraping bottom of skillet to loosen browned particles, until gravy thickens slightly (about 5 minutes). (4 servings)

Apple Slaw

4 cups finely shredded green cabbage
¼ cup low-calorie Italian dressing
  Dash of salt
⅓ cup juice drained from sweet pickles
1 unpared apple, slivered
  Dash of salt

A short while before serving, toss together all ingredients. (4 servings)

Spanish Peaches

1 30-ounce can cling peach halves
3 tablespoons dark brown sugar
1 tablespoon grated lime peel
1¾ tablespoons lime juice
⅓ cup sherry

At least 2 hours before serving, drain peaches, reserving ½ cup syrup. In small saucepan, combine peach syrup, brown sugar, lime juice, and sherry. Simmer 5 minutes. Place peach halves, flat side

156

down, side by side in a serving dish and pour the syrup mixture over them. Sprinkle peaches with grated lime peel. Refrigerate until serving time. (About 8 servings of one peach half per serving)

Stuffed Prunes

       2 cups sugar-frosted cereal flakes, crushed
       1 cup confectioners' sugar
      ⅓ cup chopped walnuts
       1 package pitted prunes (12 ounces)
       1 tablespoon lemon juice
      1½ teaspoons grated lemon rind

In a bowl, mix all the ingredients together with the exception of the prunes. Cut a slit in the side of each prune and fill with the mixture. Store tightly covered. (6 or more servings)

Chops à L'Orange

      16 center-cut loin pork chops,
              thinly sliced
      ½ cup flour
       1 teaspoon seasoned salt
       2 tablespoons butter or margarine
      1½ cups chili sauce
      1½ teaspoons prepared mustard
      1½ teaspoons garlic salt
       1 tablespoon soy sauce
      2½ tablespoons brown sugar
       2 cups orange juice

Carefully trim all obvious layers of fat from chops. In a small bag, mix together flour and seasoned salt. Toss chops, one at a time, in flour mixture and shake off any excess.

In butter or margarine, in a large and deep skillet or Dutch oven, sauté the pork chops on both sides until golden brown. Meanwhile, in a medium bowl, mix together chili sauce, mustard, garlic salt, soy sauce, and brown sugar. Stir in orange juice. Arrange chops in

157

the skillet or Dutch oven and cover with the sauce. Simmer, tightly covered, for 30 minutes. Remove cover and boil gently 30 minutes longer or until chops are tender and sauce has thickened to a nice consistency. Serve with the sauce. (8 servings)

Spicy Italian Casserole

1	small eggplant, peeled if desired
1¼	cups thinly sliced zucchini
1⅓	cups thinly sliced onions
1	cup spaghettini, broken in 3-inch pieces
3	cups canned vegetable-juice cocktail
1	tablespoon Worcestershire sauce
1	teaspoon salt
1	teaspoon garlic salt
¼	teaspoon oregano

Preheat oven to 325° F. Slice eggplant ¼ inch thick. In a 1½-quart casserole place a layer of eggplant, then a layer of zucchini, then layers of onions and spaghettini. Repeat layering until casserole is full, ending with eggplant. With fork, combine vegetable-juice cocktail, Worcestershire, salt, garlic salt, and oregano. Pour over eggplant and zucchini, then cover. Bake 1¼ hours or until vegetables are tender, placing sheet of foil, with edges turned up, on lower rack to catch any juices. Before serving, spoon some of juice in casserole over top of zucchini and eggplant. (6 servings)

Kikt Biff Med Dillsas
(Boiled Beef With Dill)

2	pounds boneless sirloin beef
1	tablespoon butter or margarine
1	10½-ounce can condensed beef bouillon
1	cup water
1	teaspoon salt
	Dash of black pepper
1	teaspoon dried dill weed
1	tablespoon cornstarch
1	tablespoon vinegar
2½	tablespoons sugar
	Parsley sprigs

About 2 hours before serving, trim away as much fat as possible from meat. Cut meat into 6 serving pieces. In butter or margarine, in a large skillet with a tight-fitting cover, brown beef well on both sides. Add beef bouillon, water, salt, pepper, and dill. Cover and simmer gently 1½ hours or until beef is tender. Drain broth from beef. Measure one cup into a small saucepan. Mix together cornstarch, vinegar, and sugar to form a smooth paste. Stir into broth and cook, stirring constantly, until thickened and smooth. Serve beef topped with this gravy. Garnish with the parsley. (6 servings, 240 calories per serving)

Breakfast in a Glass

- 1 cup skim milk
- 1 egg
- ½ teaspoon vanilla extract
- 1 cup fresh fruit

Put all ingredients into blender, cover and blend. Chill before serving. 250 calories.

Oster-Cal

- 1 egg
- 2 tablespoons corn oil
- 1¼ cups skimmed milk powder
- 3 cups water
- ¾ teaspoon vanilla extract
- Artificial sweetener

Combine all ingredients in blender. Cover and blend. Chill before serving. Divide into 3 servings for a full day's menu of about 950 calories.

Carrot-Pineapple Cocktail

- 2 cups pineapple juice
- 2 small carrots, cut in 1-inch pieces
- 1 slice lemon, ¼ inch thick
- 1 cup crushed ice

159

Put juice, carrots, and lemon into blender. Cover and blend until carrot is liquefied. Remove cover and add ice; continue blending until ice is liquefied. (3 servings, about 50 calories each serving)

Tomato Juice Cocktail

2 cups tomato juice
1 slice lemon (with peel)
1 sprig parsley
1 strip green pepper
1 stalk celery, cut in 1-inch pieces
1 slice cucumber, unpeeled
¼ teaspoon Worcestershire sauce
½ teaspoon salt
1 cup crushed ice

Put all ingredients except ice into blender container, cover and blend. Remove cover and add ice. Continue to blend until ice is liquefied. (About 3 servings, each about 35 calories)

Cold Curried Chicken Soup

3 tart apples, pared, cored, and sliced
½ large onion, peeled and sliced
1 tablespoon butter or margarine
2 teaspoons curry powder
  Salt to taste
  Freshly ground pepper to taste
3 drops red-pepper seasoning
3 cups chicken consomme or broth
1 cup dry white wine
1 cup light cream
1 cup very finely diced cooked
    chicken
  Paprika

160

Cook apples and onion in butter or margarine over low heat, stirring often, until soft. Do not let them brown. Stir in curry powder and cook 3 minutes longer. Add salt, pepper, red-pepper seasoning, chicken consomme or broth, and wine. Simmer, covered, for 10 minutes, stirring frequently.

Puree in a blender or press through a fine sieve. Chill thoroughly. Just before serving, stir in cream and chicken, then sprinkle with paprika. Serve icy cold.

Marinated Shrimps or Lobster

2 pounds large shrimps, shelled and deveined or 3 packages, 10 ounces each, frozen lobster tails
1 quart boiling water
3 bay leaves
1 teaspoon salt
2/3 cup olive oil
1/3 teaspoon dry mustard
1/3 teaspoon dried basil or thyme
1/3 cup fresh lemon juice
Freshly ground pepper to taste
Fresh dill or parsley sprigs

Drop shrimps into boiling water with bay leaves and salt; cook over low heat about 5 minutes, or until shrimps are white and opaque. Drain and cool.

If using lobster, cook, following package directions. Drain, cool, and remove meat from shells; cut into bite-size pieces. In a deep bowl (not aluminum), combine olive oil, mustard, basil or thyme, lemon juice, and pepper. Add shrimps or lobster. Cover and refrigerate at least 2 hours. At serving time, drain shrimps or lobster, reserving marinade, and arrange on a platter. Pour a little of the marinade over top. Garnish with fresh dill or parsley sprigs. (6 servings)

Spanish Shrimp Salad

1 cup olive oil
¼ cup white vinegar
¾ teaspoon grated rind of lemon
¼ cup lemon juice
1 clove of garlic, mashed
3 tablespoons capers, drained
1 teaspoon sugar
⅛ teaspoon liquid red-pepper seasoning
Salt to taste
Freshly ground pepper to taste
4 cups deveined, shelled, and cooked
shrimps (about 1½ pounds)
1 large sweet onion, peeled and
thinly sliced
Salad greens
Thin lemon slices

Combine olive oil, vinegar, lemon rind and juice, garlic, capers, sugar, red-pepper seasoning, salt, and pepper. Mix well. Place shrimps and onion slices in alternate layers in a deep bowl (not aluminum). Pour dressing over the layers. Chill, covered, 4 hours or overnight. At serving time, drain shrimps and onion. Place on a platter lined with salad greens. Garnish with lemon slices.

Chicken Escallope

1 pound boned, skinned chicken breasts
½ teaspoon salt
½ cup chicken bouillon
1½ tablespoons lemon juice
2½ tablespoons chopped parsley
1 tablespoon chopped chives
(frozen or freeze-dried)
¼ teaspoon dried leaf marjoram

Slice chicken breasts lengthwise. Place between two pieces of foil; pound with side of cleaver or rolling pin to flatten. Sprinkle with salt. In skillet, put 2 tablespoons of bouillon; add chicken and brown lightly over high heat. Add remaining bouillon, lemon juice, and herbs. Cook over moderate heat about 20 minutes, until tender. (2 servings)

Raspberry Parfait

2 10-ounce packages frozen raspberries,
   thawed
2 cups liquefied nonfat dry milk or skim milk
1 package vanilla rennet custard dessert

Drain juice from raspberries. Divide ½ of raspberries among six 5- or 6-ounce parfait glasses or custard cups. In a small saucepan, heat milk to lukewarm and remove from heat. Stir in rennet custard until completely dissolved. Gently pour ⅓ cup of custard mix down sides of each glass onto raspberries. Let stand undisturbed until firm (about 10 minutes). Top with remaining raspberries and juice. Refrigerate until chilled, *but do not freeze.* (6 servings, about 130 calories each)

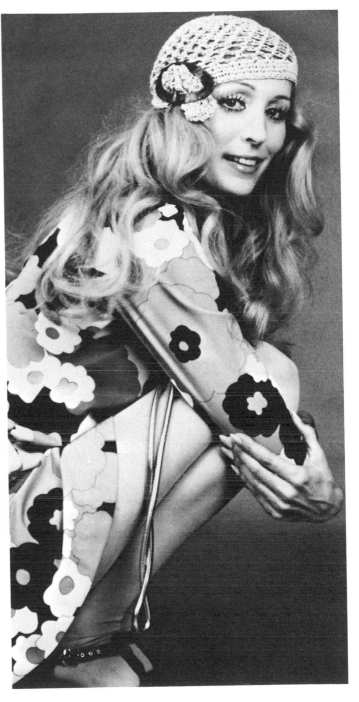

Oleda and all other models know that the style of clothes you wear can make you look slimmer or heavier. *(Photo: Steve Ladner)*

CHAPTER · 20

How to Look
Slimmer
in Ten Minutes

Midway through your diet you'll discover the new *you* who is emerging. And oh, how you'll want her to hurry up and show herself! Well, she's on her way but there's certainly no need for you to wait until the end of dieting to begin showing off. Now's the time for a sneak preview of the glamor that's to come.

There are simply dozens of ways to make yourself appear slimmer than you are, and it takes no more than the ten minutes it takes to dress. We models are adept at the business of illusion and believe me, it doesn't end with makeup and hairdo. We're something of magicians when it comes to fashion, too. So supposing you are . . .

Short-Waisted

Tanya Leveau is, but you'd never know it. And here are the magical rules she follows to create the illusion of a longer waistline:

When you wear a belt, never put it smack on the waist. Instead wear it low at the hips. Pants? Hip huggers that nestle on the hipbone are great for your figure. (How's *that* for a stylish solution to a figure

166

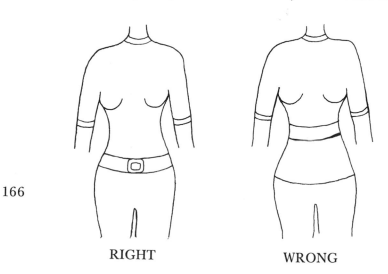

RIGHT   WRONG

problem?) Tanya almost always avoids a two-color dress, finding that one color is a delicious way of s-t-r-e-t-c-h-i-n-g the waistline.

Short

I'm forever surprised at how many of the legendary film stars are tiny when you see them in the flesh. Joan Crawford, for example, is about 5'3". And even the fabulous Marlene Dietrich isn't much taller than that. Of course, most models are tall (and some like Verushka skyscrape to nearly six feet!), and when the job demands it, they even know how to exaggerate their willowy silhouettes.

If it's more height you're after, avoid dramatic fashions that tend to wear you instead of vice versa. Choose, rather, silhouettes that feature softness in line and detail. Lightweight fabrics are fine, but quilted or stiff fabrics aren't. Very small prints and one-piece dresses are divine on the short figure and, of course, you should scale your accessories accordingly. Avoid chunky jewelry and oversized handbags.

If you're short and still rather full-figured midway through your diet, create the illusion of being further along the road of the new slim *you* by choosing vertical lines in styling. Naturally, you'll avoid a tight-waisted look, settling instead for the easy waistline that will not interrupt the vertical lines of your outfit. Dress in dark colors (black is ultra-chic, and so are various rich shades of dark brown, deep, deep wine, and deep, soft greys). A solid-color box-shaped jacket worn over a dark straight skirt is divine camouflage.

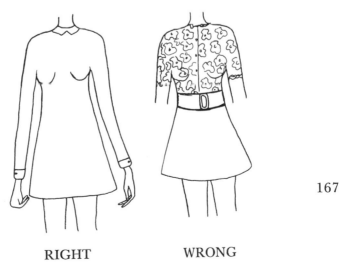

RIGHT   WRONG

167

Bosomy

Wilhelmina is, as have been some of the most famous models of all time. And since fashion designers and photographers sometimes decide against using a model when they are too conscious of her frontage, it behooves a working model to know how to draw eyes away from her ample bustline.

Eschew tight-fitting clothes at all costs. Ditto anything with "fussy" details—say, a ruffled blouse. Veer toward the more sophisticated clothes: the one-piece dress which emphasizes the vertical line (and perhaps features some fashion accent at the hem), V-shaped necklines and long rounded necklines, which are an intriguing way of drawing attention up and away from the bosom, blouses and jackets that flare gracefully at the hips, as well as anything styled along the A-line.

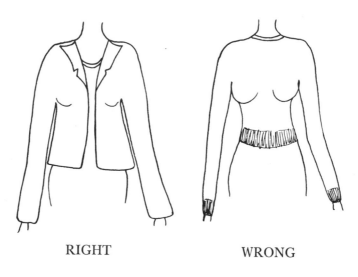

RIGHT   WRONG

Hippy

When statuesque Norma Jean Dardin weighed 140 pounds, her hips were her biggest problem. Still, she insisted on wearing slacks, and what's more she got away with it by seeing to it that her slacks were always either in solid, subdued colors or were quietly striped. And always *pocketless.* When it came to skirts, Norma Jean wore them gracefully full, for she realized only too well that a tight-fitting skirt

168

would emphasize that her hips were in need of slimming. Slight flares and A-lines are strongly recommended until your hips are exactly the size that you want them.

While I don't consider myself hippy, the bony area just above my hips is a trifle wide, so I, too, follow many of the fashion rules set down for the hippy figure. For example, I will never wear anything "extra" over my hipbones—belts, thick fabrics, and so on. In fact, I position belts either over or below this point.

Shoulder-to-shoulder detailing is a marvelous way to balance a still hippy figure (for example, a long and beautifully colored silk scarf). A wide low neckline, large collars, and bodice detail are also especially flattering. A tunic or a boxy jacket worn over pants is another neat way to cover the hip area. And once again, wearing one color is preferable to more than one color; multi-colored outfits have a tendency to cut the figure and thereby draw attention to the widest area.

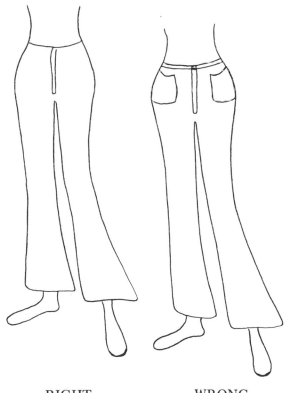

RIGHT   WRONG   169

Short-Legged

A long, leggy look is divine. And even if your legs are long and sleek, you may want to follow these tips to emphasize them.

Heather Hazell has a rather long torso and simply will never be convinced that her pretty legs are long enough, particularly for a fashion model who earns her money and fame gliding down a runway. So Heather wisely wears one color and, when possible, carries this color into her hose as well—for instance, a creamy beige suit or dress with stockings that match or almost match, and pumps that are perhaps only a few shades darker. (Marlene Dietrich, she of the gorgeous legs, almost always follows this rule, too—not that she needs to, but with legs like hers she naturally wants to draw attention to them!) Also, make a point to position your belt at your natural waistline or, if the outfit permits, higher. The Empire style is *you*. And bodice detailing will do wonders for your figure. In short, the higher your legs appear to start, the leggier you'll look.

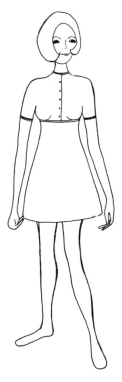

170

RIGHT

Wide-Shouldered

Avoid padded shoulders at all costs. Instead choose clothes with raglan or dolman sleeves, and narrow lapels on jackets. Wear scarves with strong vertical lines.

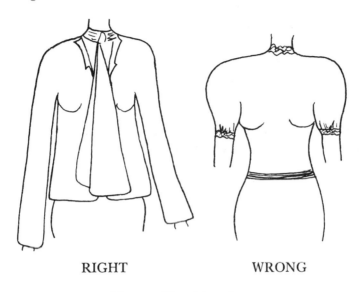

RIGHT   WRONG

Narrow-Shouldered

Bare as much neckline as fashion (and modesty) permit. Avoid balloon sleeves. Wear cap sleeves or long, narrow sleeves. Never, ever go sleeveless—that makes narrow shoulders practically disappear.

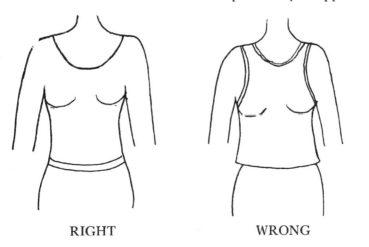

RIGHT   WRONG

171

Heavy in the Arms

Like the girl with too thin arms, you must avoid all extremes in sleeves—too tight or too loose. Instead, choose natural, soft effects.

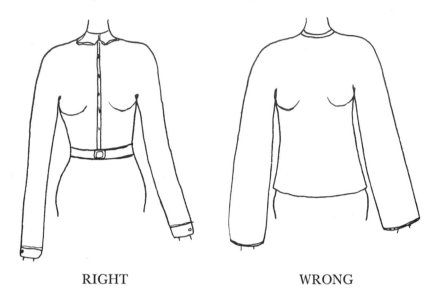

RIGHT   WRONG

Short or Plump in the Neck

The V-necklines and wide low necklines are by far the most flattering. Wear your hair up or short, and you'll seem to add inches to your neck length. Never, ever wear anything fussy at your neckline.

172

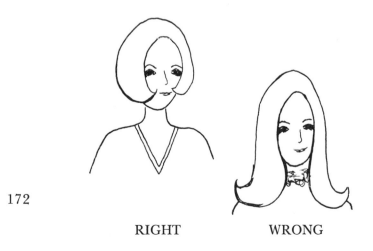

RIGHT   WRONG

Protruding in the Tummy

Avoid clothes that are tight-fitting. Avoid anything double-breasted. Avoid narrow skirts. But skirts with soft fullness or front drapery are immensely flattering.

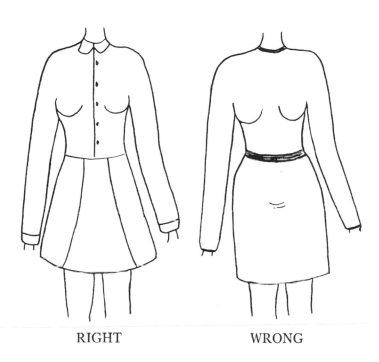

RIGHT   WRONG

173

Learn to be a make-up whiz and you'll be able to minimize imperfections and achieve nearly any look you want. Model Norma Jean Dardin loves the new natural cosmetics whipped up from such things as strawberries, lemons, and cool cucumbers.

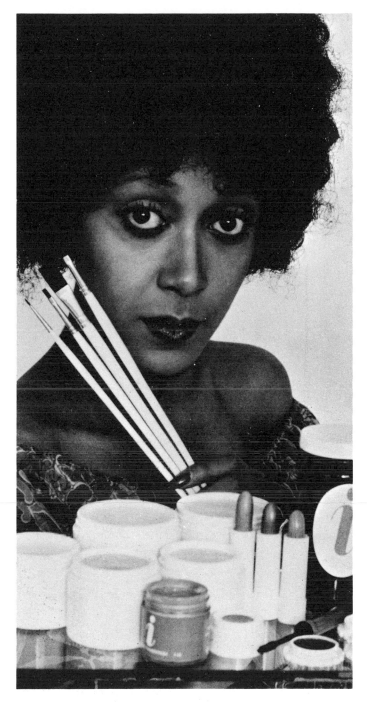

CHAPTER · 21

How to Achieve the Illusion of a Near-Perfect Face

Not even the highest paid cover girl has a perfect face. But everyone has the ability to look near-perfect. That should be good enough; a perfect face has too few surprises. And furthermore, what a sense of accomplishment (and witchery!) it gives a girl to make so-so features appear alive and glamorous. For example:

THIN LIPS. Judy Brown's lips really aren't thin, but neither are they as luscious looking as she'd like them to be. So, here's what she does.

Using a light brown or auburn eyebrow pencil (or, if you prefer, a pink lip liner pencil), she outlines the outermost part of her lips (touching the skin next to the lips slightly) and then fills in with a lipstick closest in color. For instance, a cocoa lipstick is a lovely complement to a light brown pencil. Then, Judy blends the lip rouge with her little finger, basically following her true lip shade but "cheating" just a little, making her top lip slightly higher and extending both corners a tiny bit. In the same subtle way, she makes her bottom lip appear fuller and rounder. The result is a 1920-ish mouth—curvy and a little bit pointy at the top. She's always so pleased with the result that, after blotting her lipstick, Judy uses a gleamer to highlight her lips; she puts a tiny dot at top center and two dots on her bottom lip, one on each side where the lip is fullest. Then she deftly blends in all three dots for a truly kissable look!

TOO FULL LIPS. Tanya Leveau has a voluptuous mouth that she considers too full for a petite girl. Therefore, she calls attention to her exotic eyes and plays down her lips as follows: She snubs plain lipstick, preferring a mix of lipstick and vaseline, which she makes herself. Here's the recipe. Into a skillet place an aluminum rack—the type you can buy in the kitchen department of any department store or five-and-ten. Then put about half an inch of water into the

176

bottom of the pan and place it over a *low* flame. On the aluminum rack place a flat metallic pillbox (metallic so it won't melt). When the pillbox has heated, take a leftover lipstick (or two or three leftover lipsticks of complementary colors); break off the tip and put it into the now-hot pillbox. The lipstick will melt on contact. Now, with a butter knife add a few pats of vaseline and stir with the handle of the knife. Result: a divinely colored lip gloss you can put on with a lipstick brush or pat on with your fingertips. Very subtle. Very shimmery.

Norma Jean Dardin claims a little "cheating" also works wonders. To create a thinner lip line, she suggests you start off by covering your mouth with makeup base, making sure the base is heavy enough to camouflage the outline of your mouth. Then powder your lips with whatever face powder you use. Now draw your lip line no more than a sixteenth of an inch inside your natural lip line.

ROUND FACE. Judy Brown again. Remember I told you how this very popular young model worked at shedding umpteen pounds to become more sophisticated looking? She succeeded, of course, but she also realized that no amount of healthful dieting will ever give her a hollow-cheeked Dietrich look. So clever Judy creates the *illusion* of a slimmer, high-cheekboned face, and you can, too. Here is the way:

Put a couple of dabs of gleamer at the top of each cheekbone. Next, apply brown shading cream or brown creme eye shadow (if your skin is oily, use a cake) just underneath both cheekbones, but not close to your nose. Now, blend in both gleamer and brown cream with outward and slightly upward strokes.

THIN FACE. It's possible, but not too likely, that despite a too generously proportioned figure, your face is too thin. But if that's the case, take heart. Soon your figure will be slim, and in the meantime you can add the illusion of gentle curves to your face by using a bronze blusher on the cheekbone itself for a healthy, natural look.

LONG NOSE. Not a few of the top models have noses that are a bit too long. And it hasn't kept them from popping up on the covers of

177

the most glamorous magazines! So if your nose is longer than you'd like it to be, do what these clever girls do:

Add a dab of darker foundation to the undertip portion of your nose. (Darker shades minimize too-prominent features by cutting down on light reflection.) Next, draw even more attention away from the vertical line of your nose by emphasizing the horizontal line: highlight the sides with a foundation two shades *lighter* than your natural skin tone. Of course, you blend very, very carefully for a natural look.

TOO SHORT NOSE. Naturally the trick here is to emphasize the vertical line, so now it's a lighter-than-usual foundation applied down the very center of your nose, stopping at the tip.

FLAT NOSE. Tanya Leveau points out that most Orientals have flattish noses, so this is a beauty problem she learned to solve years ago. Here are her rules, which she also recommends for black beauties who want to use them:

Keep eyebrows far apart so less shadow cuts across bridge of nose.

Mix beige and white foundations and pat the mixture on your nose bridge; this will keep the bridge from receding and will give your nose a more sculptured look.

SEMI-WIDE NOSE. That's me. Just about one inch above the nostrils—just about where the nose begins to fan out on both sides—my nose is a bit too broad. So I shade it at this point (after applying makeup base but before powdering) by using a brown eyebrow pencil on each side of my nose, then smudging it with up and down strokes.

RECEDING CHIN. Glamorous Audrey Hepburn has one. So does Wilhelmina, who claims to hate profile shots because of it, despite the fact that the editors of *Vogue* and *Harper's Bazaar* went into raptures over her profile. In any event, if you've decided your chin needs more character, here's how to add it:

With light foundation make a wide triangle over your chin. Begin it from a point just below your lower lip, and go up along your jawline to a point halfway between your chin to your ear. Blend.

UNDEFINED JAW LINE. Here's where fashion model Heather Hazell offers a tip: apply a darker shade of makeup base (or a bronze blusher) to your jawbone all the way around. Blend and powder.

SQUARE JAW. Apply a dark foundation on the outer sides of your face and jawbones. Then, start your blusher close to your nose, and blend it out and up toward your hairline and down toward your jawbone.

DOUBLE CHIN. Use a dark foundation directly below your jawbone. Blend it from ear to ear along the jawline and down under the chin line.

SMALL EYES. Cover the lids with a light foundation. Draw a very fine line with an eye liner along the upper lashes, taking care not to come quite into the inner corner of the eye. Add a line below the roots of your lower lashes, too, extending it beyond the outer corner of the eye. Use a bright-colored shadow on the upper lid, very close to the lash line.

TOO-CLOSE-TOGETHER EYES. Apply eye makeup on the outer half of your eyes. Pluck your brows so they start directly over the inner eye corners (farther away from your nose).

DEEP-SET EYES. Use white or off-white eye shadow from lash line to brow. Add a very thin line of eye liner.

Joanne Dusseau skis, rides horseback, and bicycles all over town, and I predict that with that sports schedule (one she can stay with for life)—and that mental attitude—she'll never have to fret about poundage.

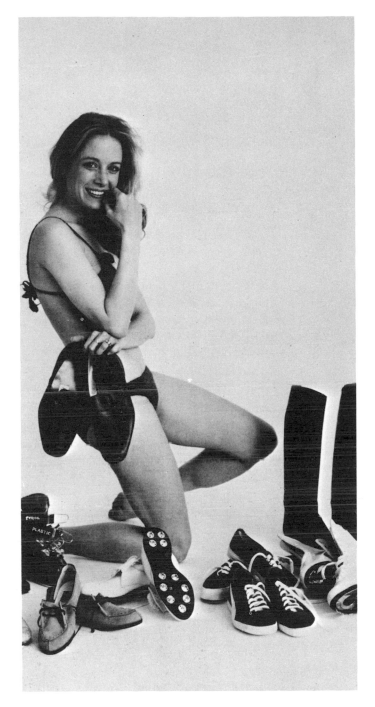

CHAPTER · 22

How to Stay Slim Forever

The Coed No-Age-Limit Exercises

We Americans are a tremendously sports-minded people; we're also very gregarious—a combination that finds us very team-oriented when it comes to sports. All of which is just fine while we're young, and particularly when we're still in school. But what happens when we mature and are left more or less to our own devices? All too often we become spectators, watching and cheering somebody else exercise.

I think it's high time we all discovered at least one independent sport; by *independent* I mean one that doesn't require being part of a team. If possible it should be a sport you can enjoy all by yourself and one that won't be out of bounds to you even when the number of candles start concealing the icing on your birthday cake.

SWIMMING is one of these no-age-limit exercises that's particularly wonderful since you can enjoy it year round. My son began swimming when he was barely 4 years old, and I often wonder why I waited so long to teach him; I've seen infants of six months and less happily paddling in a pool. Swimming exercises *every* part of your body from the neck right down to the ankles. It stretches and firms your entire body. Furthermore, it helps relieve tension, for it just isn't possible to swim and worry at the same time.

No wonder many models make a point of swimming five or six times a week. One girl became even more of a swimming enthusiast when she spied actress Kitty Carlisle in the pool each and every time she went for a dip. And anyone who has seen this vivacious lady on television will understand why the model was so impressed. Miss Carlisle has the slim, graceful figure of a girl: tiny waist; slender, youthfully rounded arms; trim hips. Yet Kitty Carlisle was a singing star in the films of the early thirties!

182

HORSEBACK RIDING is a delightful exercise that whittles away at the hips. Have you ever seen a hippy cowboy? Of course not. You may not have the opportunity to ride horseback, but if you do—take advantage of it. Many models vacation at dude ranches just for the opportunity to reduce their hips while riding in the intoxicatingly fresh, dry desert air.

BICYCLING gets a hearty vote from models as both a sleek exerciser and a practical mode of transportation in a city like New York, where bumper-to-bumper traffic isn't at all uncommon. Cycling is a fabulous hip-whittler that also does equally flattering things for your waistline, legs, and derriere. Judy Brown, whose legs are quite literally her fortune, is a bicycling enthusiast. She has her "wheel" stashed in her apartment for regular weekend excursions in Central Park, where our mayor has very thoughtfully closed the roads to automobile traffic at certain times. Model Joanne Dusseau rides her bicycle all over town, and Marianna Heiser took up biking to help her sons with their suburban paper route, loved the exercise so much that she kept right on pedaling long after she stopped delivering papers.

Like swimming, bicycling is soothing for the nerves and, according to the most learned physicians, it's an exercise heartily recommended for the heart. Dr. Paul Dudley White, who treated President Eisenhower after his first heart attack, has stated that he'd like to put everybody on bicycles. In many small cities in Europe, where the cost of an automobile is prohibitive, bicycles are still the chief mode of transportation. Here in affluent America we are, I think, victims of our automobiles. Why not get a bicycle for yourself? It could be one of the best investments you'll make this year!

SKIING is slimming . . . soaring . . . sensational. I love it! My husband and I ski practically every weekend in the winter, and by the time I've slipped off my cap and gloves and snuggled up to the fireplace after an entire day outdoors in the sun and snow, I tingle from head to toe—especially around the waist, hips, and legs. All that bending and twisting on the slopes, particularly once you've mastered the parallel turn and the short stem christie, is a positive

183

beauty treatment for the figure! You have only to look at the skiers in their après-ski stretch pants to see for yourself how this classic sport tightens and firms those spots where too many women have a tendency to bulge and spread. And again, this is a no-age-limit sport you can enjoy solo or with your entire family.

GOLF was once considered a masculine sport. And quite frankly, I suspect that was what first attracted me to it. (I was single, and what girl doesn't find interesting a sport that abounds in men?) Well, let me tell you that it's a superb female sport, too—great for the arms, tummy, and waist, and, if you bypass a cart and walk from tee to tee, it does wonders for your legs, too. Today, of course, golf is a unisex sport. If you didn't actually see Ruby Keeler on stage in "No, No, Nanette," making her comeback after some 40 years, you probably have seen her on one or more television shows: still pert, with a wedding band waistline and those simply gorgeous legs! Charming Ruby is a near champion golfer and is, I think, as exciting an advertisement for golf as Kitty Carlisle is for swimming.

TENNIS, anyone? If I had my way, that famous old line (first spoken onstage by, of all people, Humphrey Bogart) would read, Tennis *everyone*! Steve and I play in spring and summer. I'm not as good as I'd like to be, but I feel great after a game. (Any game that has LOVE in its score should be taken up by married couples, don't you agree?) Again, here's a lively sport that has you racing, reaching and s-t-r-e-t-c-h-i-n-g. I wager that tennis burns up more calories per hour than any other sport. And remember those marvelous old-time newsreel shorts of King Gustavus V of Sweden? A lanky giant of a man who played a smashing game of tennis until he was past 90! So you see, it's a lively sport that helps keep its practitioners lively, too. Dinah Shore and Ginger Rogers are two tennis buffs. Both are, chronologically speaking, many years past girlhood, but their svelte figures simply haven't paid any attention to the calendar years.

WALKING—a sport? I think so. I regard walking, like swimming, as a superb all-around exercise. It's a natural, anybody-can-do-it kind of exercise that is particularly beautifying to your legs and complex-

184

ion—provided, of course, that you walk *briskly.* Models are all great walkers, for often we simply can't get a cab, can't wait for a bus, and so we walk. And we walk fast—we're always in a rush! I realize it's simpler to walk in a city than it is in a suburb, where often a sidewalk peters out and a highway takes over. If that's your terrain, why not do your walking further out in the country? Drive there, park your car, and get out and *walk.* Make it a brisk walk of exploration. If you have a dog, take him along and let him race. Involve your husband or boyfriend in a weekend walking program. Remember, walking helps develop circulation in the heart muscle, and heart specialists recommend it, like bicycling, as a heart disease preventive.

Walking is great for children, too. It's never too soon, in my opinion, to introduce children to physical activities they can enjoy all their lives. Competitive team sports are fun and important, but they are temporary. We tend to outgrow teams as we mature. Walking, on the other hand, is a *lifetime* sport.

Some people get even more fun from their walking by using a pedometer. It gives them a positive sense of accomplishment. I don't carry a pedometer, but I know that I walk an average of 3 miles every day. So what gives me my sense of accomplishment? A statement by Dr. Harry J. Johnson, author of *Creative Walking,* to the effect that not only is walking one of the best ways to achieve and maintain a slender figure, but a brisk daily walk will also increase your sense of well-being and your sex appeal. Understandable, then, that Gaylord Hauser urges his followers to "Walk and walk and walk—with long, long steps—everywhere, every day of your long life!"

DANCING—an exercise? You know it is! A *fabulous* exercise, particularly since the discotheque was born and the energetic New Wave dances swept into sight. I vividly recall cosmetic queen Elizabeth Arden, then almost 80, enthusing over the Twist as "a perfectly wonderful exercise for the waistline!"

I love to dance, and many models I know study dancing as a form of exercise. In fact, most cities have schools that teach dancing not only as a lovely means of self-expression, but also as an exquisite way to a slimmer, firmer, more responsive body.

The YWCA here in Manhattan gives budget-priced lessons in *Tai Chi Chuan,* an ancient, nonstrenuous exercise that is a particularly graceful way of keeping fit. The basis of it is the figure eight, around which are woven some 108 forms—all performed upright and with absolutely no strain. Your body is constantly in motion but it's more like *slow* motion, blending a serene sense of fluidity with proper breath control. It may sound complicated, but it is as simple as it is natural. And it works wonders. You may have seen *Tai Chi Chuan* performed on television's "Today Show" a few years ago. I found it fascinating.

Milton Feher's School of Relaxation and Dance is also in Manhattan, and as the name suggests, his teachings, too, will not leave you in a state of complete exhaustion. A former ballet dancer, the whippet-slim Mr. Feher teaches you the art of relaxation *before* he guides you over to a ballet bar and starts you limbering up. The result is a form of dance exercise that trains your body to take maximum pleasure in performing the simple acts of standing, sitting, and walking with all the grace of a true ballerina.

The Carnegie Hall Studios next door to Carnegie Hall house some of this city's most creative and colorful people. Charlotte Hess is one of them—a doll-like Viennese with shiny dark hair in a coronet braid, sparking eyes, and gorgeous legs. Her studio is one of those miraculously high-domed affairs with mirrored walls, and a skeleton hanging from a ribbon in one corner. Sound ghoulish? Not at all. Miss Hess teaches all forms of social dancing, but before a student so much as takes the first step, she learns to stand straight. Proper posture is essential to graceful dancing. And that's where the skeleton enters the picture, with la Hess using it for demonstration purposes. To her, dancing is a form of balanced walking. So when a student completes a course with Charlotte Hess, she'll not only have the steps of a dance down pat, but she'll also have a more thorough knowledge of and respect for her body.

What if you live in a smaller city or town and don't have such a feast of dance courses to select from? Well, unless you live in a truly mini-sized hamlet, you probably have at least one dance school. If you don't, however, there are innumerable dance books available that are beautifully illustrated and simple to follow. Folk dancing, for example, is tremendously popular with many sophisticated

186

models. Not at all surprising either, since so many young Americans today are looking to our past for comfort and a sense of belonging. And folk dancing, with its ethnic roots and traditional steps, is such a vigorous and happy way to exercise.

But whatever kind of dancing you prefer, do it with all your heart, and you'll find it not only an exciting exercise but a tonic for your personality, too. Dancing regularly puts bloom in your cheeks, sparkle in your eyes, and a spring in your step at any age.

CHAPTER · 23

The Models'
Potpourri
of Beauty Tips

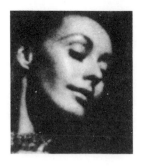

ALEXA ADAMS—Height: 5'10" Weight: 125 pounds. Alexa eats two meals a day (favorites are Chinese food and any fish) and refrains from snacks between meals. For exercise and enjoyment she attends ballet classes twice a week, rides horses on the weekend, and takes long, long walks.

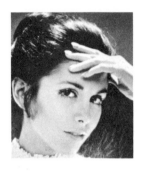

DANA CARROLL—Height: 5'8" Weight: 112-110 pounds. Dana told me that the diet that works best for her is as follows: "I limit my carbohydrate intake to 20-25 grams per day but allow myself all the protein and fats I want because they are filling. Certain low-carbohydrate vegetables are allowed, such as lettuce, celery, tomatoes, green beans, broccoli, and asparagus—also all meats and cheeses, except prepared meats such as liverwurst and salami. Have one glass of milk a day and a piece of fruit (orange, grapefruit, melon). Use margarine, vegetable oils, vinegar, and mustard, but mayonnaise, ketchup, and salt should be used sparingly." In order to have nice nails, Dana has a manicure each week and keeps polish on them at all times. She also takes gelatine pills and water-soluble vitamin A. If she wants to look especially tall and thin, she wears a monochromatic outfit, such as navy slacks and a navy sweater. This creates a long, lean look because there is no break in color.

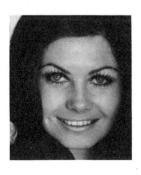

PAT BARRIE—Height: 5'6" Weight: 112 pounds. Pat's system for losing weight makes a lot of sense. She says: "Cut out potatoes, noodles, rice, and all bread. Cut down on salt and butter. Eat carrots, salads, and drink club soda. Instead of having snacks, I dreak tea with lemon and bouillon with celery stalks. Within one week I can lose five pounds, and if I need to lose more I exercise more to use up more calories. I take vitamin E and iron for extra energy, and eat wheat germ, half a grapefruit, one egg, and tea for a good breakfast." For muscle tone, Pat does a combination of dance exercises and any other stretching exercises, concentrating on the waist, hip, and leg muscles. Her nails were very weak, so she takes Knox Gelatine and keeps her nails at medium length. Pat enjoys all sports, plus photography, cooking, sewing, reading, and dancing (modern and jazz). Since she is short for a model, she wears clothes that give the illusion of height, like pantsuits and fabrics that cling to the body, accenting her waist with interesting belts.

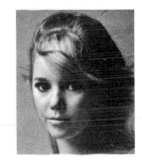

KATHY JACKSON—Height: 5'8½" Weight: 110 pounds. Her secret way to lose: "I pretend that I've already eaten what I crave most and I fill up on a lot of liquids such as juice, tea, and water." Kathy has weighed as much as 130 pounds, so her secret method must be doing some good. Also helpful is the fact that she lives in a seventh floor walk-up apartment. She attends Columbia University several nights a week and reads whenever she can find extra time.

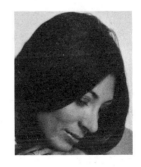

JANIE JENNINGS—Height: 5'8½" Weight: 118-120 pounds. Although Janie's choice of foods is good for any diet (filet mignon, lobster, salads, shrimp, etc.), she finds it necessary to use her will power. If she eats too much one day, she will eat much less the next. Janie feels that in order to keep her skin in the "pink of condition," she must drink plenty of juices, and she scrubs daily with an almond and honey preparation. To keep it smooth, she uses Nivea cream. When I asked her about her hobbies, she gave me this list:

cooking (especially experimental recipes)
dancing (every chance I get—great exercise)
sewing (every now and then I get creative)
motorcycles (for a little excitement)
traveling (whenever I can)
my dog (who runs me ragged)
My Man (who should have been at the top of this list!)

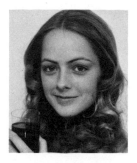

ROXANNA VLADY—Height: 5'7'' Weight: 118 pounds. Because Roxanna has to watch her weight constantly, she eats a lot of fruits and vegetables and dances a lot. She also does the typical exercises for slimming her arms and waist. For thin hair with split ends, she finds that trimming often and using Neutrogena shampoo helps to keep it looking nice. Roxanna wants to become an actress, and her love of dancing and interest in people may help her to reach her goal. In sports, she has an adventurous spirit and will try anything. "Be natural" is her motto.

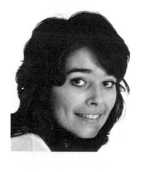

VICTORIA DIAZ—Height: 5'8¾'' Weight: 118 pounds. Victoria shies away from full meals, and snacks most of the time on carrots, celery, grapefruit, 7-Up, and clam chowder. When she has the urge to eat, sometimes she runs out to the country and sits in a field alone until the craving for food leaves. Her weight must be watched constantly, because she has gone as high as 132 pounds and as low as 101 pounds. When it's really necessary, she will go on a special diet of fluids for two days, then eat only raw vegetables, meats, and fluids until she gets down to the desired weight. She rides a bicycle at least once a week and walks to all appointments whenever possible. For fat on the upper-inner thigh, she does the leg-slapping exercise. (Sit on the floor with arms behind you and knees bent, one foot 6 inches forward of the other, then open and close legs as hard as possible.) Victoria loves to dance; she tries to go places where she can dance on the weekends. She was born in Lima, Peru, and finds people from other countries fascinating.

MARY RIECHERS—Height: 5'8½" Weight: 120 pounds. Mary likes all vegetables, salads, veal, ice cream, mushrooms, all fish, tea, and shortbread. Her average daily calorie intake is from 1,500 to 1,800. Her favorite dishes include mushroom salad, and a salad of spinach, mushrooms, and bacon served with oil and vinegar. She finds a strict diet of fish and salads helps her lose weight extremely fast. For lunch she will have only tea or bouillon; and for breakfast, yogurt. To protect her nails, she wears rubber gloves and uses plenty of hand lotion, also a nail strengthener cream and nail polish at all times. Mary never uses soap on her face, but swears by Propa Ph. Drinking fat-free milk and yogurt helps her teeth, skin, and nails. For trim thighs, she does the following exercise daily: lying on her side, she brings her leg straight up, then to the side, repeating ten times for each leg. Mary is a registered nurse and works at it part time. She also rides horses and goes on canoe expeditions. The ecology movement is of great interest to her.

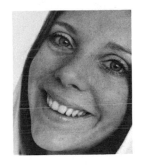

JOANNE DUSSEAU—Height: 5'8" Weight: 112 pounds. Since Joanne's weight can vary from 133 to 97 pounds, she eats only one big meal a day (usually breakfast) and snacks about two or three

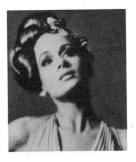

times a day on apples, avocados, yogurt, and cheese. To keep trim, she does general exercises to limber up each morning and rides her bicycle all over New York City. Modeling is her special interest because it earns her "bread." She is an actress and studies voice and dance, going to classes every night. She also engages in many sports for exercise.

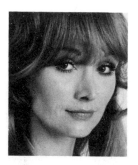

VERNICE GABRIEL—Height: 5'7½'' Weight: 120 pounds. Vernice had to redevelop her taste for food because she had always loved rich and spicy foods and all desserts, creating a constant weight problem. Now she maintains her weight by eating a well-balanced diet of high-protein and low-carbohydrate foods such as prime ribs of beef (rare), steak tartare, or any broiled meats, leafy green salads (she loves spinach salad and Caesar salad), eggs, and green vegetables, and she has lost all taste for desserts. Because she is very active through the day, she finds little time to sit down for breakfast or lunch, so she snacks on carrot and celery strips, grapefruit, tomatoes, and shrimp cocktail. She says that she is much healthier and happier now. Her secret way to lose weight is to plan a big party, "then knock yourself out with setting the atmosphere and organizing all the details yourself." Or she will go on a sports kick—ice skating, roller skating, riding horses, and bicycling. Her favorite hobby is "being a woman." She says she is happiest when she is pleasing her husband and making her children happy. She also enjoys interior decorating, designing, and sewing, "exploring the Flea Market for hidden values," and traveling. Because she has full hips, she wears A-line dresses and flared-bottom slacks to minimize them and give her a leaner look.

194

JACQUI CARR—Height: 5′8″ Weight: 117 pounds. Jacqui has no special diet, although she loves Japanese food. Her weight and figure are maintained by her keeping active and practicing yoga. For snacks she munches on apples and raisins. One tip she gives is to drink water frequently through the day; it curbs the appetite and adds no calories. Jacqui perfers the soft, natural look in makeup, *sans* false eyelashes. She likes to travel and meet interesting people.

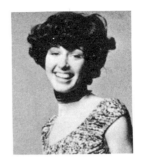

RANDE HAGUE—Height: 5′7½″ Weight: 112 pounds. A well-balanced diet is Rande's approach to eating. This gives her the energy to enjoy such outdoor sports as horseback riding, swimming, water skiing, etc. Indoors, she has been developing her talent for interior decorating, because she has a fourteen-room house in the country to practice on. To keep her hair at its best, she shampoos daily, as it has a tendency to get very oily.

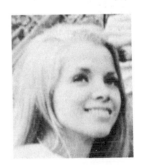

SHARRON WRIGHT—Height: 5′7″ Weight: 110 pounds. Sharron *loves* to cook, but eats only brunch and dinner each day. She has been on a diet for the past ten years and feels she will be forever. Since her weight has gone as high as 130 pounds, she refrains from eating any snacks between meals. She sticks to a high-protein, low-carbohydrate diet with plenty of meats, fish, cheese, green vegetables, and fresh fruit. She finds that riding her Honda is great for bouncing the fat off, especially on the New York City streets! She also finds that her figure keeps trim because of her *being* a model, because of all the walking and the strength needed to carry those heavy portfolios which are so essential to the profession. To keep her hair soft and

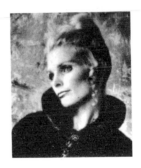

lovely, she uses a good conditioner, namely Revlon's Flex. For soft, smooth skin, she feels you must apply a good body lotion or baby oil in the morning and at night. She has found that her nails become harder and healthier when she is in France, and attributes this to the hard water they have and the mineral water that she drinks there. Sharron has won prizes for her art, and she and her partner have won national championships in ice skating. She also enjoys swimming, dancing, horseback riding, and "playing pool."

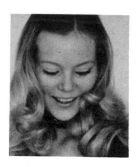

TAFFIE WELLS—Height: 5'7" Weight: 105 pounds. When Taffie has to lose weight, she eats vegetables, fruits, and meat cooked on the broiler, and she eliminates all starchy foods. Also, Juicerator drinks are a favorite of hers. Here is a recipe she has for a delicious low-calorie salad:

Guacamole

2   medium-sized ripe avocados
1   large tomato
1   tablespoon chopped white onion
2   ounces French dressing
1   teaspoon finely chopped serrano chilies
½   teaspoon coriander seed, crushed
    Dash of tabasco sauce
    Juice of ½ lime
    Salt and pepper to taste

Whip all ingredients together until you get a smooth consistency. Serve with tortilla.

She has solved the problem of thin hair, which seems to be a dilemma for her. After washing, bend over so that the hair hangs down in front of you and brush while drying with a blower-type dryer. This makes the hair appear fuller.

BARBARA CARRERA—Height: 5'8" Weight: 118 pounds. Barbara loves food, but eats one meal a day most of the time, and will not snack between meals. Too much acid will create a problem for her skin, but she is an advocate of organic vitamins (especially vitamin E) and *clean* skin. Occasionally Barbara has to crash diet, using the liquid diet or low-carbohydrate diet. Her fingernails are her major beauty problem, so she applies several coats of nail-building polish over and under the nails to protect them. Her interests are playing the guitar and piano for relaxation or for friends, art, languages, and entertaining people from different nations. She also likes the challenge of learning new things; otherwise she becomes bored.

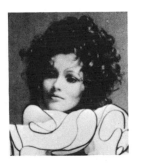

JILL KELLY—Height: 5'7" Weight: 103 pounds. Jill loves to cook, so she must watch what she eats to maintain her present weight. (When she went to college, she gained about 20 pounds.) She has adopted a routine of dieting through the week, and "the sky's the limit" on the weekends. Because she has a tendency to be bottom-heavy, she must spot-exercise as follows: Lie on the back, bend the legs and bring the knees to the chest, keeping them together. Roll them from the waist to the left side, then back to the chest. Legs straight down, then repeat the same on the right side. Jill also does sit-ups to firm the stomach muscles. These exercises, she says, should be done at least 25 times each night before going to bed. Most of Jill's favorite foods are all protein, but the side dishes can be a diet problem. She has a variety of effective diets, so that she doesn't get bored with eating the same foods. One week she will eat a lot of vegetables and little meat. Then she will try the "Stillman's Diet." With both diets, she advises drinking plenty of water. Jill loves sports such as swimming, tennis,

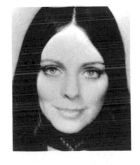

197

and horseback riding, and enjoys reading and decorating. She dresses according to her mood, sometimes sophisticated, tailored, sporty, or just fun and "a sloppy kind of neat." She sews suede and leather accessories for a hobby.

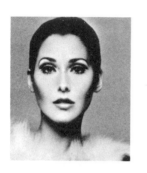

MERLE LYNN BROWNE—Height: 5'7" Weight: 103 pounds. Merle feels that eating slowly and chewing your food well are aids to reducing. She loves all salads and food well prepared. She feels that if you have to lose weight, you must consider it an individual problem and not follow the latest fad diet; if one doesn't work, try another. Merle is interested in people as individuals and finds it a challenge to get through the barriers we create to avoid showing the real us.

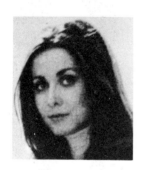

BEVERLY LAKE—Height: 5'10" Weight: 125 pounds. Eggs, shellfish, dried fruit, cheese, pickles, celery, pineapple, cottage cheese are some of Beverly's favorite foods. Because she constantly has to watch her weight, she sticks to high-protein foods, and eats a half grapefruit before every meal. Her hair is very thin and long, so she uses Thicket, which thickens and conditions the hair. For dry skin, she uses Kenneth's Skin Drink Lotion, and if the skin breaks out, she uses Thera-Blem. For stronger nails, she advises using Revlon's Wonder Nail. Beverly has a B.A. in mathematics and loves to relax by playing tennis and skiing.

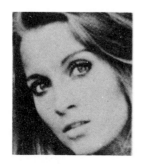

GUNILLA PARK—Height: 5'9½" Weight: 130 pounds. Gunilla goes to health clubs for swimming and saunas wherever she happens to be in the world. Her favorite food is steak and she snacks on cheese, fruit, and salads with seafood. When her skin gives her trouble, she avoids sweets (especially chocolate). Her interests are reading in different languages, psychology, and astrology. A fashion trick for looking slimmer is to wear black and to choose clothing that is designed with a long look.

ERIKA TOTH—Height: 5'6½" Weight: 108 pounds. Erika says that she loves to cook but has disciplined herself never to snack between meals. Although she eats three meals a day, she burns off most of the calories by being very active and refraining from eating desserts. Because her hair is very oily, she must wash it every day unless there is no important event happening; then she will use a dry shampoo. Erika is an excellent figure skater, which helps to keep her trim, and she also enjoys other sports such as swimming, skiing, and walking. She has learned that some colors don't look as good on her as others, and no matter how good the style might be, she won't buy an item for her wardrobe unless the color does something for her.

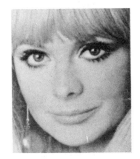

ELEANOR POOLE—Height: 5'10" Weight: 122 pounds. Among the foods Eleanor enjoys eating are roast beef, steak, salads, veal, lobster, and oranges. Because these foods are high in protein and low in carbohydrates, she doesn't have to watch the calories. However, if she finds herself even five pounds overweight, she will cut down on the amount she eats. To keep her skin at its best and prevent acne, she washes her face three times a day and applies a moisturizer to prevent dry skin. Once a week she will apply an oatmeal mask, which also helps to prevent any acne problems with her skin. When she feels a need for exercise,

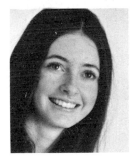

199

she does sit-ups, toe-touches, and handstands, although playing tennis and dancing give her plenty of exercise. When Eleanor was 6, she started dancing lessons and continued for four years. She still does a lot of dancing and has now combined acrobatics with it, so she has very little need for extra exercise. She enjoys reading whenever she can find the time. In fashion she will wear only what suits her and will not fall victim to fads.

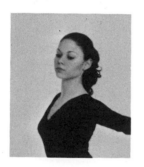

DARIA—Height: 5'6" Weight: 102 pounds. Daria's plans after finishing high school are to become a professional ballet dancer. She is now attending two classes a day at the School of American Ballet. Ballet is the most strenuous exercise there is; but even though she has no need for weight watching or typical exercises, she limits herself to a substantial breakfast and lunch. Her "secret" for losing weight and maintaining it is "don't eat dinner."

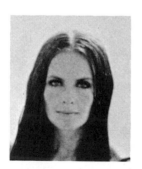

ROSEMARY HOWARD—Height: 5'9" Weight: 117-120 pounds. Eating food all week that is high in protein and indulging on the weekends has worked satisfactorily for Rosemary. For snacks she will have Swiss cheese, shrimp, or Jello. Rosemary says: "Grapefruit is a good way to break down fat," and "I find I can maintain a diet much longer if I give myself little treats every few days." Because Rosemary believes that rest, a peaceful outlook, and having a good time are the best beauty tips, she has worked out a routine for herself. "Get eight hours' sleep, have a face cleaning once a month, a facial weekly, walk a lot, wash your hair every other day, have a manicure every second week. After I put myself together in the morning, I try to spend the rest of the day thinking about

other things than myself." Rosemary is going to
Columbia to get her B.A. She is interested in writing, painting, photography, making stained glass
windows, and has written a cookbook that is un-
published as yet.

SHIRLEEN TUCKER—Height: 5'7" Weight: 115
pounds. Because her hair is very dry, Shirleen visits
the hairdresser every ten to fourteen days for a
complete treatment and conditioning. She never
sets her hair, keeps the scalp oiled and brushes it
often. One of her assets is her clear, smooth skin
which she cleanses thoroughly each day. Shirleen
hopes to be a fashion coordinator or buyer some-
day and has been getting good experience by teaching charm in the city schools and a modeling
school. Her hobbies include reading, cooking, wine
and cheese tasting, music (collects jazz albums),
painting with acrylics, and collecting antiques and
oriental art objects.

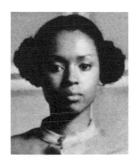

RENEE DAVID—Height: 5'8" Weight: 120
pounds. Renee's favorite foods are lamb, shellfish
(shrimp and lobster), salads, and cheese, and since
she eats everything in moderation, she has no problem controlling her weight. She spends her time
taking care of her two children and yet finds the
time to sew, knit, decorate, and work on developing her voice and talents for acting.

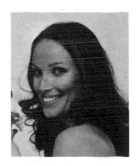

AIMEE LIU—Height: 5'6" Weight: 100 pounds.
Aimee has always had to control her weight because she loves food (any kind). She told me that
she thinks about food all the time and has to keep
active in order not to eat too much. Presently, she

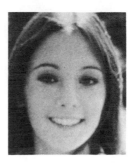

is concentrating on a vegetarian diet and feels that uncreamed cottage cheese is the most nutritious and least fattening food. She feels excrcise is essential and generally walks over a mile each day— even more in the city. Aimee's main concern is school, which she enjoys very much. Modeling is just a means of earning money for her college education. The only beauty problem she has encountered so far is the circles under her eyes, but she conceals these by using Ultima Cream Concealer by Revlon.

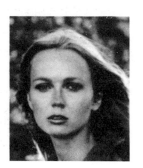

PENNY JAMES—Height: 5'6½" Weight: 106 pounds. Penny watches her weight constantly and tries to limit her calorie intake to 1,700 per day. She eats eggs, fish, cheese, vegetables, and broiled meats. She told me her object is not to lose weight, but to maintain it, and when she gets five pounds over her desired weight she eats only high-protein foods and stops using butter, breads, and gravy dishes. Penny has a good system for exercising that makes it more pleasurable. "To maintain a good figure, I put music on that I like, stand in front of a full-length mirror, and do dance exercising. This is always done on my toes—anything goes as long as it looks graceful. Also try a lot of stretching exercises."

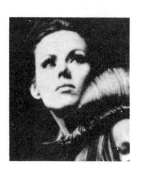

INGRID DRECHSLER—Height: 5'8½" Weight: 118 pounds. Ingrid has her eating plan regulated in such a way that she has no problem with weight watching. She eats lightly and sticks to foods such as salads, fruits, leafy green vegetables, shellfish, and tuna fish. If her figure gets just a little out of line, she cuts down the quantity of food and does a few toning exercises. Ingrid loves walking in the woods with her dog, horseback riding, bicycling, tennis, and cooking.

CHRIS PALMER—Height: 5'10½" Weight: 122 pounds. Chris says that "activity is the best weight watcher," and "if you gain a little, you must be prepared to be hungry a few days, and having a strong, mental outlook helps." Chris is still going to school, but finds time to write, sew, paint, play guitar, and do needlepoint from her original designs. For muscle tone and a general relaxed feeling, she does stretching exercises. For snacking, she will have a cup of tea or a glass of white wine.

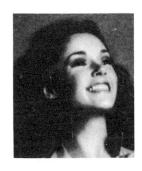

CARMEN—Height: 5'7½" Weight: 120 pounds. Carmen's secret for maintaining her weight is: "Simply eating what I like in moderate portions, eating one meal a day, not snacking." Her nails used to keep splitting in layers, until she found that constantly keeping nail polish on them holds them together. Also, she finds that wearing rubber gloves and eating protein (eggs and milk) helps keep them healthy. She keeps them squared-off so they will be less likely to snap. Cleansing the face is a very important part of her daily schedule. Using Georgette Klinger products (well-known among the models), she gives herself a weekly facial, then uses creams and lotions to keep the skin conditioned daily. Carmen has one major problem which she related to me as follows: "Being a black person in a white world, I've had to imitate what I couldn't duplicate—straight hair. One of my earliest child-hood memories is my mother washing my hair one day, me sleeping with a "bushy" head (now known as a "full Afro" or "natural") and then spending the next day crying while my mother straightened my hair with a hot comb and then curled it with a hot curling iron and oiled my poor aching head. As I grew up, I learned to handle the instruments of torture by myself, and when I entered the business world my first regular expense was weekly trips to

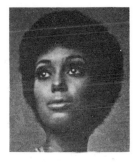

the hairdresser. Then, miracle of miracles, cream releasers were introduced. At the same time, I became a model and the condition and line of my hair became even more important—so important that I was having my hair straightened every four to six weeks, in addition to using hot rollers or a curling iron on it, and coloring it once a month. This is not a compatible combination for healthy hair. This routine went on for years, and for some reason my hair did not suffer severe damage. It was probably due to the fact that I carefully conditioned my hair every week and after each straightening. I do remember being burnt and having raw sores on my scalp until I was fortunate enough to find a hairdresser who knew how to handle straighteners, and more important, who cared. The solution to such severe maltreatment of my hair and scalp was "doing what comes naturally"—an Afro (or natural, if you will). No more burning hair or scalp; no more closets full of conditioners, sprays, rinses, dyes, special shampoos; and more time to myself, since hair care is no longer an ordeal. I still use cream rinses and conditioners, so my hair is healthier than it's ever been before." Carmen has found that an all-around diet of milk products and other protein foods is good for her nails and hair, and avoiding carbonated drinks, chocolate, and fried food is beneficial to her skin. Since excess weight tends to settle in her hips and thighs, she walks as much as possible, does exercises that concentrate on those areas, and finishes with stretching exercises so that the muscles become elongated instead of bunched up. Carmen loves to cook, sew, and watch old movies on television.

PAMELA HECHT—Height: 5'7" Weight: 100-105 pounds. Pamela eats one main meal a day and a

light protein lunch, with no snacks in between.
This allows her to splurge during that one meal
with dishes like lasagna, beef Bourguignon, baked
Alaska, lemon meringue pie, or baked potato with
sour cream. Pamela is big on salads and grapefruit.
Since she washes her hair every day, she uses
Clairol's Condition each time instead of a cream
rinse. Her dermatologist formulates her makeup list
because she is allergic to all products on the
market. As an astringent she uses a mixture of
alcohol and ether. She uses Piz Buin suntan lotion
when exposed to the sun, because her skin is ultra-
sensitive. Pamela takes dance lessons twice a week,
plays tennis, water skis, and rides horses, so she
feels at this point there is no need to do special
exercises to keep trim. She also writes poetry and
short stories.

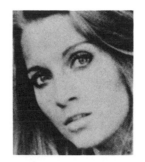

YOLANDE CATHARINE FLESCH—Height: 5'9"
Weight: 118 pounds. Her favorite foods are Chinese
food, brown bread with cheese, cantaloupe, and all
Dutch food. She has a tendency to gain weight
when she is bored—she can't think of anything else
to do but eat. On a tedious location job there is no
relief except for the lunch break, during which she
stuffs herself. This is partly because she has asso-
ciated food with rest from work. To keep from
thinking about food, what she does is think of
something exciting to do. She also takes a long
look at fat ladies and tells herself, "I never want to
look like them." She has no special diet, but uses
an extra thrust of will power when she realizes that
she is losing control. She respects her body. She
also enjoys doing the yoga exercises and has one
for her bust, stomach, and thighs. These exercises
make her feel loose, yet tighten the muscles.
Yolande feels that eight to nine hours of sleep each
night are a must for her. Her main interest is traveling, which her job gives plenty of opportunity to

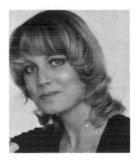

do. She has already been on an around-the-world location job, and enjoys anything that involves being outdoors during the summer.

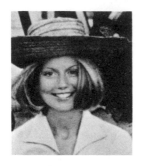

SALLY-ANN VANCLIFFE—Height: 5'8'' Weight: 117 pounds. At age 15, Sally-Ann weighed 176 pounds. Unhappiness causes her to overeat, but she has found the answer to her problem. "The best remedy for anyone is to fall in love. I was at my happiest and thinnest while under the spell of a certain Frenchman." She also supplements this remedy with trips to the gym and ballet exercises. Having been a dancer, she also frequents discothèques.

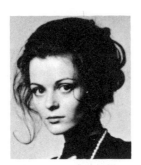

LAUREL LEE—Height: 5'6½'' Weight: 100 pounds. It took about a year of eating liquid diet foods, vegetables, and fruits to reduce from 123 to 105 pounds. Laurel used to have a problem maintaining her weight, but after practicing the diet routine for so long, she has become more disciplined. The only problem she now has is bad posture, for which she has an exercise. Stand next to a wall with feet about 6 inches from the wall. Bend knees until back is flat against the wall, then slowly straighten up, keeping back against the wall. This flattens the tummy and gives you better posture, making you taller. To give the illusion of being taller, Laurel wears close-to-the-body clothes and a "small-head" hair style. Laurel claims this is her secret way to lose weight: "When I see I've put on a pound or two, I cut out all snacks and meals except dinner for one or two days. The first day is a little hard, but I find I eat less dinner than if I had snacked during the day. I get filled up with less because my stomach shrinks. I can go back to eating normally, but I will eat less because my appetite is reduced and I'm satisfied with less." Because her hair is so long, it tends to dry out and split at the ends, so she washes her hair with a mild acid-balanced shampoo. She feels alkaline soaps are drying. Once in a while she will soak the bottom of her hair in olive oil before washing. Because her skin is very sensitive and has a tendency to dry out, she uses Redken soap, which cleans the skin without irritating it.